Acute and Reconstructive Burn Care, Part II

Editors

FRANCESCO M. EGRO
C. SCOTT HULTMAN

CLINICS IN PLASTIC SURGERY

www.plasticsurgery.theclinics.com

July 2024 • Volume 51 • Number 3

ELSEVIER

1600 John F. Kennedy Boulevard ● Suite 1800 ● Philadelphia, Pennsylvania, 19103-2899

http://www.theclinics.com

CLINICS IN PLASTIC SURGERY Volume 51, Number 3
July 2024 ISSN 0094-1298, ISBN-13: 978-0-443-12923-0

Editor: Stacy Eastman
Developmental Editor: Anita Chamoli

Clinics in Plastic Surgery (ISSN 0094-1298) is published quarterly by Elsevier Inc., 360 Park Avenue South, New York, NY 10010-1710. Months of issue are January, April, July, and October. Business and Editorial Offices: 1600 John F. Kennedy Blvd., Suite 1800, Philadelphia, PA 19103-2899. Periodicals postage paid at New York, NY and additional mailing offices. Subscription prices are $576.00 per year for US individuals, $100.00 per year for US students/residents, $631.00 per year for Canadian individuals, $703.00 per year for international individuals, $100.00 per year for Canadian students/residents, and $305.00 per year for international students/residents. For institutional access pricing please contact Customer Service via the contact information below. To receive student/resident rate, orders must be accompanied by name of affiliated institution, date of term, and the *signature* of program/residency coordinator on institution letterhead. Orders will be billed at individual rate until proof of status is received. Foreign air speed delivery is included in all *Clinics* subscription prices. All prices are subject to change without notice. **POSTMASTER:** Send address changes to *Clinics in Plastic Surgery*, Elsevier Health Sciences Division, Subscription Customer Service, 3251 Riverport Lane, Maryland Heights, MO 63043. **Customer Service: 1-800-654-2452 (US and Canada). From outside of the United States and Canada, call 314-447-8871. Fax: 314-447-8029. E-mail: JournalsCustomerService-usa@elsevier.com (for print support); JournalsOnlineSupport-usa@elsevier.com (for online support).**

Reprints. For copies of 100 or more of articles in this publication, please contact the Commercial Reprints Department, Elsevier Inc., 360 Park Avenue South, New York, New York 10010-1710. Tel.: +1-212-633-3874; Fax: +1-212-633-3820; E-mail: reprints@elsevier.com.

Clinics in Plastic Surgery is covered in *Current Contents, EMBASE/Excerpta Medica, Science Citation Index, MEDLINE/PubMed (Index Medicus), ASCA,* and *ISI/BIOMED.*

Contributors

EDITORS

FRANCESCO M. EGRO, MD, MSc, MRCS
Associate Professor, Departments of Plastic
Surgery and Surgery, Deputy Chief of Plastic
Surgery UPMC Mercy, Associate Director of
UPMC Mercy Burn Center, Director of Burn
Reconstruction, Director of Medical Student
Education, Associate Program Director
Integrated and Independent Residency,
University of Pittsburgh Medical Center,
Pittsburgh, Pennsylvania, USA

C. SCOTT HULTMAN, MD, MBA, FACS
Chair, Department of Plastic and
Reconstructive Surgery, WPP Plastic and
Reconstructive Surgery, WakeMed Health and
Hospitals, Raleigh, North Carolina, USA;
Campbell University, Buies Creek, North
Carolina, USA; Department of Plastic and
Reconstructive Surgery, Johns Hopkins
University, Baltimore, Maryland, USA;
Campbell University School of Osteopathic
Medicine, Lillington, North Carolina, USA

AUTHORS

ARYA ANDRE AKHAVAN, MD
Plastic Surgery Resident, Division of Plastic
and Reconstructive Surgery, Department of
Surgery, Rutgers New Jersey Medical School,
Newark, New Jersey, USA

MARIO ALESSANDRI BONETTI, MD
Research Fellow, Department of Plastic
Surgery, University of Pittsburgh Medical
Center, Pittsburgh, Pennsylvania, USA

SIGRID A. BLOME-EBERWEIN, MD
Associate Professor, Department of Burn
Surgery, University of South Florida
Morsani College of Medicine, Lehigh Valley
Health Network, Allentown, Pennsylvania,
USA

MARTIN R. BUTA, MD, MBA
Postdoctoral Clinical Research Fellow, Division
of Plastic and Reconstructive Surgery,
Massachusetts General Hospital, Harvard
Medical School, Department of Plastic,
Reconstructive, and Laser Surgery, Shriners
Hospitals for Children, Boston, Massachusetts,
USA

MATTHIAS B. DONELAN, MD
Associate Professor, Department of Surgery,
Harvard Medical School, Chief of Staff,
Emeritus, Shriners Hospitals for Children -
Boston, Visiting Surgeon, Division of Plastic
and Reconstructive Surgery, Massachusetts
General Hospital, Boston, Massachusetts,
USA

FRANCESCO M. EGRO, MD, MSc, MRCS
Associate Professor, Departments of Plastic
Surgery and Surgery, Deputy Chief of Plastic
Surgery UPMC Mercy, Associate Director of
UPMC Mercy Burn Center, Director of Burn
Reconstruction, Director of Medical Student
Education, Associate Program Director
Integrated and Independent Residency,
University of Pittsburgh Medical Center,
Pittsburgh, Pennsylvania, USA

MARK D. FISHER, MD, FACS
Director, Bayview Adult Burn Center, Associate
Professor (Pending Academic Review),
Department of Plastic and Reconstructive
Surgery, The Johns Hopkins University School
of Medicine, Johns Hopkins Burn Center,
Baltimore, Maryland, USA

C. SCOTT HULTMAN, MD, MBA, FACS
Chair, Department of Plastic and
Reconstructive Surgery, WPP Plastic and
Reconstructive Surgery, WakeMed Health and
Hospitals, Raleigh, North Carolina, USA;
Campbell University, Buies Creek, North
Carolina, USA; Department of Plastic and
Reconstructive Surgery, Johns Hopkins
University, Baltimore, Maryland, USA;
Campbell University School of Osteopathic
Medicine, Lillington, North Carolina, USA

YING C. KU, DO
Plastic Surgery Resident, Department of
Surgery, Campbell University School of
Osteopathic Medicine, Lillington, North
Carolina, USA

WILLIAM NORBURY, MD, MBBS
Associate Professor (Pending Academic
Review), Department of Plastic and
Reconstructive Surgery, The Johns Hopkins
University School of Medicine, Johns Hopkins
Burn Center, Baltimore, Maryland, USA

REI OGAWA, MD, PhD, FACS
Professor, Department of Plastic,
Reconstructive and Aesthetic Surgery, Nippon
Medical School, Tokyo, Japan

NELSON S. PICCOLO, MD
Chief, Division of Plastic Surgery, Pronto
Socorro Para Queimaduras, Goiânia, Goiás,
Brazil

DEBRA ANN REILLY, MD, FACS, FABA
Professor Emeritus, Department of Surgery
(Plastic), University of Nebraska Medical
Center, Omaha, Nebraska, USA

J. PETER RUBIN, MD, MBA, FACS
Chair, Department of Plastic Surgery,
University of Pittsburgh Medical Center,
Pittsburgh, Pennsylvania, USA

**SHANMUGANATHAN RAJA SABAPATHY,
MS, MCh, DNB, FRCS (Ed), FAMS, Hon
FRCS (Glas), Hon FRCS (Eng), Hon FACS,
DSc (Hon)**
Chairman, Department of Plastic Surgery,
Hand and Reconstructive Microsurgery and
Burns, Ganga Hospital, Coimbatore, Tamil
Nadu, India

**R. RAJA SHANMUGAKRISHNAN, MBBS,
MS, MRCS, DNB**
Consultant Plastic Surgeon, Department of
Hand, Reconstructive Microsurgery,
Faciomaxillary and Burns, Ganga Hospital,
Department of Plastic Surgery, Hand and
Reconstructive Microsurgery and Burns,
Ganga Hospital, Coimbatore, Tamil Nadu,
India

ANNA WHITE, MD
Resident Physician, Department of Surgery,
University of Nebraska Medical Center,
Omaha, Nebraska, USA

Contents

 Video content accompanies this article at http://www.plasticsurgery.theclinics.com.

In recent decades, advances in surgical anatomy, burn pathophysiology, surgical techniques, and laser therapy have led to a paradigm shift in how we approach burn scars and contractures. Scar excision and replacement with uninjured tissue, which predominated burn scar treatment for much of the 20th century, is no longer appropriate in many patients. A scar's intrinsic ability to remodel can be induced by reducing tension on the scar using various techniques for local tissue rearrangement. Often in combination with laser therapy, local flaps can optimally camouflage a burn scar with adjacent normal tissue and restore a patient more closely to their preinjury condition.

Rei Ogawa

Hypertrophic scars arise from burn injuries because of persistent inflammation in the reticular dermis. Several risk factors promote this chronic inflammation. One is tension on the burn wound/scar due to surrounding skin tightness and bodily movements. High estrogen levels and hypertension are also important systemic risk factors. Thus, to prevent burn wounds from developing into hypertrophic scars, it is important to focus on quickly resolving the reticular dermal inflammation. If conservative treatments are not effective and the hypertrophic scar transitions to scar contracture, surgical methods such as Z-plasty, full-thickness skin grafting, and local flaps are often used.

Sigrid A. Blome-Eberwein

In this article, an array of new developments in burn care, from diagnosis to postburn reconstruction and re-integration, will be discussed. Multidisciplinary advances have allowed the implementation of technologies that provide more accurate assessments of burn depth, improved outcomes when treating full-thickness burns, and enhanced scar tissue management. Incorporating these new treatment modalities into current practice is essential to improving the standard of burn care and developing the next generation of burn wound management methodologies.

The hand is commonly affected in thermal injuries. Hand burns account for 39% of all burns and they are involved in 34% of instances when the total body surface area of a burn exceeds 15%. Inadequate or inappropriate treatment could result in significant morbidity. The ultimate integration of a burn patient into the society largely depends on the functionality of the hands. Hence, it is important to reduce complications by providing good care during the acute stage.

Children are disproportionately affected by burn injuries. Differences between adult and pediatric burns range from epidemiologic characteristics to pathophysiological considerations, which vary between different age subgroups. All these factors must be considered in each phase of burn care. This article reviews the most important aspects of the management of a pediatric burned patient starting from the acute through reconstructive phases.

Reconstruction of burns in the head and neck region is challenging. This is because it must achieve both functional reconstruction and esthetic reconstruction. Local flaps are best for minor defects, particularly in the case of deep burns, because they bear the correct texture and color. However, for large deep burn wounds, simple grafting or small local flaps will not produce satisfactory results. It is also crucial to assess the extent and depth of reconstruction that is needed throughout the face-neck-anterior chest region, and to make the choice between techniques such as Z-plasty, skin grafting, super-thin flaps, and free flaps.

Acute burn reconstruction involves intricate strategies such as skin grafting and innovative technologies, addressing challenges in coverage and minimizing donor site morbidity. Despite being rarely used, flap reconstruction becomes necessary when critical structures are exposed, offering robust coverage and reducing complications. However, free flaps in acute burns face challenges, including a higher failure rate attributed to hyperinflammatory states and hypercoagulability. Surgical optimization strategies involve careful timing, patient preparation, and meticulous postoperative care. In delayed burn reconstruction, free flaps proved effective in functional and aesthetic restoration, with low flap loss rates and minimal contracture recurrence. Prefabricated and prelaminated flaps emerged as a solution for complex cases, ensuring the best functional and aesthetic possible outcomes in challenging facial burn reconstructions.

Scars commonly give rise to unpredictable, potentially irritating, cutaneous complications including pruritis, folliculitis, and pigment changes. These problems can be self-limiting and are prevalent in many burn cases, although their expression varies among individuals. A better understanding of the presentation, risk factors, and pathophysiology of these long-term sequelae allows for more comprehensive care of burn survivors.

Burn-related chronic neuropathic pain can contribute to a decreased quality of life. When medical and pharmacologic therapies prove ineffective, patients should undergo evaluation for surgical intervention, consisting of a detailed physical examination and elective diagnostic nerve block, to identify an anatomic cause of pain. Based on symptoms and physical examination findings, particularly Tinel's sign, treatments can vary, including a trial of laser therapies, fat grafting, or nerve surgeries (nerve decompression, neuroma excision, targeted muscle reinnervation, regenerative peripheral nerve interfaces, and vascularized denervated muscle targets). It is essential to counsel patients to establish appropriate expectations prior to treatment with a multidisciplinary team.

Regenerative therapies such as fat grafting and Platelet Rich Plasma (PRP) have emerged as new options to tackle burn-related injuries and their long-term sequelae. Fat grafting is able to promote wound healing by regulating the inflammatory response, stimulating angiogenesis, favoring the remodeling of the extracellular matrix, and enhancing scar appearance. PRP can enhance wound healing by accelerating stages including hemostasis and re-epithelization. It can improve scar quality and complement fat grafting procedures. Their cost-effectiveness, minimal invasiveness, and promising results observed in the literature have made these tools as therapeutic candidates. The current evidence on fat grafting and PRP in acute and reconstructive burns is described and discussed in this study.

CLINICS IN PLASTIC SURGERY

Dedication

Acute and Reconstructive
Burn Care: Part II

*To my wife, Alessandra, and pillar of strength, your love and unwavering
support have been my rock during my journey in the wonderful
world of surgery.
To our children, Sofia and Matteo, who are the light of my life and bring
me so much joy and purpose each and every day.
I dedicate this issue to all of you, with all the gratitude and love that a
husband and father can offer.*

Francesco M. Egro

To my wife, Suzanne, and children, Chloe, Hank, and Timothy,
who inspire me every day to be a better person and
to make the world a better place.

C. Scott Hultman

Clin Plastic Surg 51 (2024) ix
https://doi.org/10.1016/j.cps.2023.12.003
0094-1298/24/© 2023 Published by Elsevier Inc.

Preface

Acute and Reconstructive Burn Care: Part II

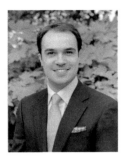 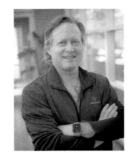

Francesco M. Egro, MD, MSc, MRCS   C. Scott Hultman, MD, MBA, FACS

Editors

Burn injuries pose one of the greatest challenges to health care professionals worldwide, requiring a multidisciplinary approach for optimal patient care. We are constantly reminded of the sheer resilience of the human spirit in the face of unimaginable pain and adversity experienced by these patients. It is with great passion and dedication that health care professionals strive to make a difference in the lives of those who have faced the inferno of acute burn injuries. This issue is dedicated to all the exceptional members of the burn team that deliver such incredible care with empathy, compassion, and unwavering commitment to our patients' well-being.

The field of burn surgery encompasses a wide range of knowledge and skills, from initial assessment and resuscitation to wound management, reconstructive procedures, and long-term rehabilitation. It is a field in constant evolution through research and innovation. This two-volume issue of *Clinics in Plastic Surgery* aims to serve as a comprehensive updated guide for burn surgeons and health care providers involved in the care of burn patients. In compiling this issue, our goal was to bring together a collection of expert insights and practical information that would not only address the fundamental principles of burn surgery but also provide valuable updates on emerging techniques and advancements in the field. Each article offers a comprehensive overview of the subject matter, supported by evidence-based approaches. Our aim is to provide readers with a clear understanding of the principles, techniques, and challenges involved in burn surgery, enabling them to deliver optimal care to burn patients and improve outcomes. We recognize that burn surgery is a dynamic and evolving field, with ongoing advancements in research and technology. Therefore, we have included articles that delve into the latest innovations and future directions in burn care, ensuring that readers stay abreast of the latest developments and are inspired to contribute to the progress of this field.

We hope that this issue serves as a valuable resource for burn surgeons, plastic surgeons, trauma surgeons, intensivists, nurses, therapists, and all health care professionals involved in the care of burn patients. It is our sincere hope that the knowledge shared within these pages will contribute to the advancement of burn surgery and, ultimately, lead to improved outcomes and quality of life for burn survivors.

Finally, we would like to extend our heartfelt gratitude to all the incredible contributors from all over the world, who have dedicated their time

Clin Plastic Surg 51 (2024) xi–xii
https://doi.org/10.1016/j.cps.2024.02.004
0094-1298/24/© 2024 Elsevier Inc. All rights reserved.

and expertise to make these issues possible. Their commitment to the field of burn surgery is commendable, and we are grateful for their contributions.

Francesco M. Egro, MD, MSc, MRCS
Departments of Plastic Surgery and Surgery
UPMC Mercy Burn Center
Burn Reconstruction
Medical Student Education
Integrated & Independent Residency
University of Pittsburgh Medical Center
Pittsburgh, PA, USA

C. Scott Hultman, MD, MBA, FACS
WPP Plastic and Reconstructive Surgery
WakeMed Health and Hospitals
Raleigh, NC, USA
Campbell University
Buies Creek, NC, USA
Department of Plastic and Reconstructive Surgery
Johns Hopkins University
Baltimore, MD, USA

E-mail addresses:
francescoegro@gmail.com (F.M. Egro)
chultman@wakemed.org (C.S. Hultman)

The Art of Local Tissue Rearrangements in Burn Reconstruction: Z-Plasty and More

Matthias B. Donelan, MD[a,b,c],*, Martin R. Buta, MD, MBA[a,b,c]

KEYWORDS

• Burns • Burn care • Thermal injury • Burn reconstruction • Burn surgery
• Local tissue rearrangement • Z-plasty

KEY POINTS

• Advances in surgical anatomy, burn pathophysiology, surgical techniques, and laser therapy have led to a paradigm shift for which the optimal approach for improving many scars is no longer scar excision.
• Hypertrophic and contracted burn scars are ideal reconstructive material: they are autologous, in the right location, and can be rehabilitated.
• Local tissue rearrangement leverages a burn scar's ability to remodel and blend in with adjacent normal tissue.
• The direction of the incision in a burn scar is just as important as the scar's location and the technique used to revise it.
• Local tissue rearrangement avoids morbidities associated with regional and distant flaps and skin grafts.

 Video content accompanies this article at http://www.plasticsurgery.theclinics.com.

INTRODUCTION

Burn scars have the potential to become patients' most valuable reconstructive anatomy after sustaining burn injuries. The art of local tissue rearrangement enables that potential to be realized and includes all the ways that the resulting scars can be revised and treated to help restore patients as much as possible to their preinjury state. It is helpful to think of burn scars as valuable assets with good qualities rather than something bad that would best be removed. Scars are autologous tissue in the right location and when revised properly, they blend well into the adjacent tissue because they are the same. In addition, scars today can be rehabilitated with lasers and laser-assisted drug delivery (LADD) to a degree that could not have been imagined 50 years ago. Using the existing scars for a patient's reconstruction eliminates the need for donor site iatrogenic injuries. It is impossible to return a patient to their preinjury state while adding donor site deformities. The quality of the final outcomes obtained by local scar tissue rearrangement is limited only by the imagination, diagnostic skill, experience, and technique of the surgeon.

[a] Plastic, Reconstructive, and Laser Surgery, Shriners Hospitals for Children, 51 Blossom Street, Boston, MA 02114, USA; [b] Division of Plastic and Reconstructive Surgery, Massachusetts General Hospital, 51 Blossom Street, Boston, MA 02114, USA; [c] Harvard Medical School, 25 Shattuck Street, Boston, MA 02115, USA
* Corresponding author. Department of Plastic, Reconstructive, and Laser Surgery, Shriners Hospitals for Children, 51 Blossom Street, Boston, MA 02114.
E-mail address: mdonelan@mgh.harvard.edu

Clin Plastic Surg 51 (2024) 329–347
https://doi.org/10.1016/j.cps.2024.02.010

This counterintuitive concept has been part of the development of the art of local tissue rearrangement for the past 170 years. Modern plastic surgery really began with the profound advances in local tissue rearrangement made possible by the development of general anesthesia in 1846 and local anesthesia in 1884.[1] Before anesthesia, there were only limited examples of surgical treatment for burn scars and contractures. Local tissue rearrangement was rare because of pain and the difficulty of performing delicate procedures without anesthesia. Patients with burn injuries were forced to live with severe deformities and significant disabilities for which there were no treatments.

Once anesthesia became available, local tissue rearrangement proliferated as surgeons strove to improve outcomes for burn patients. Multiple techniques were devised and used, building on the preanesthesia work of J.C. Fricke and Thomas Mutter during the early 19th century.[2] (Figs. 1 and 2). Many of the innovators in these early plastic operations recognized the value of preserving scar tissue. Stewart McCurdy first described the double sliding flap Z-plastic in 1898 (Fig. 3).[3] The two flaps created by the Z-incision were allowed to shift places by sliding. McCurdy later wrote

In dealing with the treatment of cicatrices resulting from burns the prime object is to preserve tissue. In no instance should any portion of the cicatricial band be removed.

The bands should be so severed as to permit their sliding upon themselves, or they should be permitted to gap where a skin flap can be adjusted.[4]

Significant advances were made in the Z-plasty and other local scar revision techniques by the beginnings of the 20th century. The first double flap transposition Z-plasty, reported by Berger in 1904, was used to reconstruct an axillary burn contracture. He described the technique as an "autoplasty by dividing the web into 2 and interchanging the flaps."[5] The importance of preserving patients' scar tissue and using it to achieve improved outcomes was a generally accepted concept. This thinking, however, was dramatically changed by the genius and innovations of Harold Gillies. Based on his extensive World War I experience, Gillies advocated for the excision of scars from trauma and burns, and replacement with uninjured skin from other areas of the patient's body, including distant tissue transferred by using the new technique of tubed pedicled flap transfer. Gillies believed that scar tissue was a bad thing and expressed his opinion forcefully. He wrote in 1920:

The simplest operation in plastic work is the excision of scars. This is important, not only from the cosmetic point of view. Apart from actual loss, no factor so impedes function as does scar tissue, whether by hampering

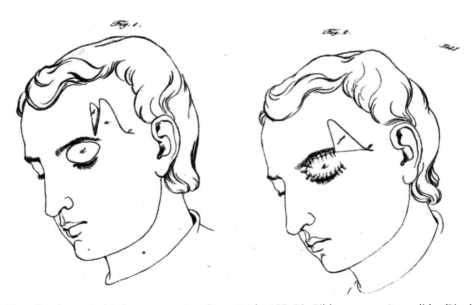

Fig. 1. Fricke's flap for periorbital reconstruction. (*From* Fricke JCG. Die Bildung neuer Augenlider (Blepharoplastik) nach Zerstörungen und dadurch hervorgebrachten Auswärtswendung derselben. Hamburg; Perthes & Besser. 1829.)

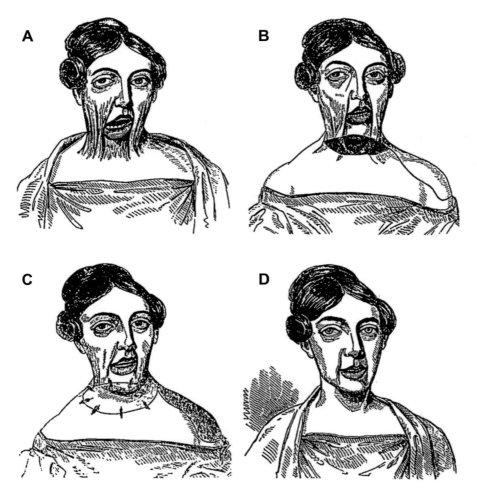

Fig. 2. Mutter's reconstruction. (*A*) Burn scar contracture of the neck. (*B*) Contracture release. (*C*) Inset of mastoid-occiput-based shoulder flap. (*D*) 12 months postop with no contracture evident in the flap. (*From* Mutter TD. Cases of deformities from burns, relieved by operation. Am J Med Sci 1842;4:66–90.)

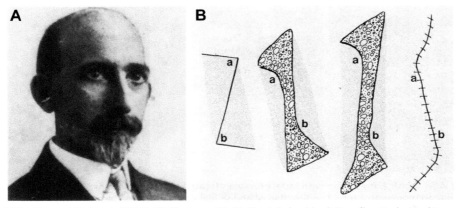

Fig. 3. (*A, B*) Dr. Stewart McCurdy (1859–1931) at age 50. McCurdy's double sliding flap Z-plastic. (*From* Borges AF. Historical Review of Z-Plastic Techniques. Clinics in Plastic Surgery. 1977;4(2):207–216.)

mobility or by the constriction of tubular organs, such as blood vessels and ducts. The general aims in scar excision are: 1) Liberation of fettered tissue 2) Restoration of contour. In either case it is essential that all the scar be excised. It is remarkable to what extent a deformity will recur if only a small amount of scar escapes. In unfavorable subjects it may be that the scar must be excised a second or even a third time before a presentable appearance is effected.[6]

Sir Harold, often described as the father of modern plastic surgery, had immense influence and his concept of scar excision and resurfacing rapidly gained increasing popularity. Many surgeons, inspired by his seminal work, as well as his negative attitude toward scar tissue, came to believe that scar excision and closure with undamaged flap skin would yield more favorable results than by locally rearranging scars or replacing them with skin grafts.[2] In 1920 he reported the case of a British Army soldier whose facial burn scars were excised and replaced with a tubed pedicle flap carried on his wrist **(Fig. 4)**.[6,7] The result shows significant improvement but armed with the retrospection scope it is informative to review this case. The linear, hypertrophic scars would have been ideal for local tissue rearranging with Z-plasties. The majority of the skin excised was unscarred. The flaps are a little inadequate and resulted in a lateral and upward contracture of the left oral commissure. The flap tissue is beardless and different in color and texture.

Gillies' thinking about scar tissue was widely accepted. John Staige Davis published an article in *Annals of Surgery* in 1931 in which he wrote, "It is a good plastic principle to remove all scar tissue before attempting any sort of reconstruction and this should be carried out whenever possible."[8] In the same article, however, Davis also recognized the potential benefits of burn scar tissue.

As we use the Z-type incision, the scar is not removed, but the contraction is relieved by the transposition of flaps, which are usually composed of scar or scar infiltrated tissue, in such a way as to break the line of scar pull. It is difficult to realize how much permanent relaxation can be secured by the use of scar infiltrated tissue, and this type of incision, until one is familiar with the procedure and its possibilities.[8]

There was still recognition by thoughtful plastic surgeons that scar tissue could play a powerful reconstructive role when "one is familiar with the procedure and its possibilities."

Sir Harold Gillies' attitudes dominated burn reconstructive thinking for most of the 20th century. Surgeons, aided by an improved understanding of surgical anatomy, better skin grafting methods and devices, and the introduction of more advanced techniques, such as microsurgery, were enabled to perform the excision of increasingly larger areas of burn scarring and closing the resulting defects with ever larger and more

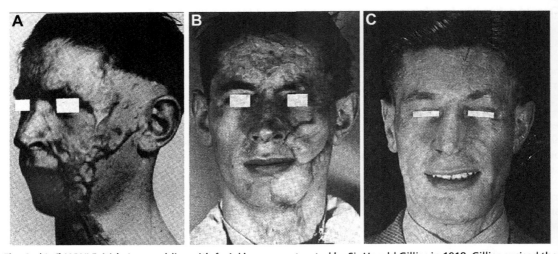

Fig. 4. *(A-C)* WWI British Army soldier with facial burn scars treated by Sir Harold Gillies in 1918. Gillies excised the scars and replaced them with a tubed pedicle flap of abdominal skin transferred by attaching it to his wrist. (*From* Gillies, H. D. (1920). Plastic Surgery of the Face Based on Selected Cases of War Injuries of the Face Including Burns with Original Illustrations. p.369–371. United Kingdom: H. Frowde.)

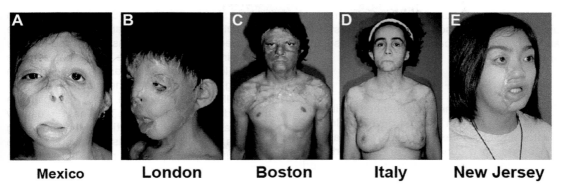

Mexico   London   Boston   Italy   New Jersey

Fig. 5. (A–E) Many burn scar excisions and flap closures result in a grotesque appearance.

complicated flaps. The ultimate example of this aggressive approach is the excision of severe facial burns and their replacement with a face transplant. Such aggressive operations can result in remarkable benefits but can also easily result in patients having complications, severe donor site deformities, and postoperative appearances that are clearly not normal.[9,10] It is essential that the results of burn reconstruction surgery make patients clearly better, not just deformed in a different way (Fig. 5).

When burn scars are rearranged and rehabilitated, they blend well into the surrounding tissues because they are fundamentally the same as the surrounding tissues. Making local flaps with and within the scar tissue uses the borders of the scars to gradually blend them into the normal. This presents an obscured image to an observer and serves as camouflage blurring the transitions from abnormal to normal. The irregular colors and textures of the scars make them less conspicuous than reconstructions done with uniform, scarless, distant flaps, which have a completely different color and texture. All of these factors help camouflage the rehabilitated scars and make them less noticeable than flaps or grafts. Facial burn scars treated with local scar tissue rearrangement and lasers show essentially normal facial expression unlike thicker distant flaps that serve as an insensate mask. All of these factors are why it is valuable to use the patient's own scar tissue whenever possible.

Perhaps the most important part of the art of local tissue rearrangement in burn scar reconstruction is knowing when it is appropriate and when the nature and extent of the scarring are too great to be reconstructed by local tissue rearrangement alone. When there is an absolute loss of tissue that requires replacement with vascularized flaps, then that is clearly indicated. Mistakes can easily be made by choosing one technique

when it is inadequate for the deformity or by choosing another which is excessive and causes iatrogenic harm. If flap tissue is required, then obviously it is the correct choice but the vast majority of the scars encountered among burn patients are superficial. That is exactly why advances in local tissue rearrangement and improved rehabilitation of burn scars have greatly helped scars achieve their potential as an asset for burn reconstruction.

The 21-century has seen a paradigm shift in how we approach scars. The revolutionary concepts of selective photothermolysis and fractional thermolysis spawned the development of lasers that can induce tissue remodeling and regeneration in scars.[11–14] Fractional ablative lasers and laser-assisted drug delivery (LADD) can also rehabilitate and improve hypertrophic and contracted scars. Laser therapy decreases tension in scar tissue and local scar rearrangement decreases tension as a primary outcome. Using both modalities creates a powerful synergy that has become standard of care in facilities which are capable of providing both forms of treatment.[15–19] Rehabilitating a patient's own injured skin in its native location can produce results that are superior to those achieved using flaps from distant sites. There is nothing like the original skin in its original location, even if it is less than perfect. Local scar tissue and scar-infiltrated tissue flaps, often in conjunction with laser therapy, can provide the optimal means for improving scar elasticity and morphology and camouflaging the rehabilitated tissues. Burn scar excision today should be employed as a last resort rather than the first step in virtually every burn reconstruction operation which was common practice 50 years ago.

Local tissue rearrangement is fundamental to scar revision. Developing an effective strategy for treating scars involves both art and science, requiring an understanding of scar pathophysiology, skin tension, scar assessment, aesthetics, and the various surgical techniques and laser therapies available.

CLASSIFICATION OF BURN SCARS

Every burn scar is unique, influenced by its etiology and the milieu in which it develops. In 2002, Mustoe and colleagues reported a scar classification based on a consensus of 12 experts from Europe, North America, and Australia.[20,21] A modified version of that classification for burn scars includes the four categories listed below (Table 1).

RELAXED SKIN TENSION LINES AND LANGER'S LINES

Skin possesses an intrinsic tension that tends to widen the border of a wound. The force vector manifests when a rounded wound opening becomes elliptical. Although skin tension exists in every direction for most of the body, it is maximal in one direction.

For many years, Langer's lines, proposed by Karl Langer in 1861, have been the most commonly referenced skin tension lines, though they apply to cadavers with rigor mortis, not living subjects. Langer determined the lines by puncturing the skin in cadavers with a rounded awl and connecting the long axes of elliptical wounds (Fig. 6).[22-24] A.F. Borges introduced the term relaxed skin tension lines (RSTLs), which exist in living subjects. These lines are not readily visible in relaxed skin but appear as ridges and furrows when pinching the skin (the ridges and furrows are the longest and most easily produced when pinching at right angles to the lines). RSTLs typically follow natural wrinkle lines, especially in the head and neck (Fig. 7A). The lines are usually at right angles to the orientation of the underlying muscles (Fig. 7B). The edges of wounds that are predominantly oriented at right angles to the RSTLs appear more widely spaced than wounds oriented along the RSTLs. This phenomenon plays a critical role in determining the direction of elective incisions: they should be made to align as closely as possible with RSTLs in order to achieve the most functional and aesthetic scar.[25-27]

SCAR ANALYSIS

Every scar has a story that warrants investigation. A detailed history and physical examination are critical to understanding a scar's history, etiology, evolution, and prior treatment, if applicable. The failure of previous interventions to achieve an acceptable outcome requires an understanding of what led to the suboptimal result. This step can help refine the treatment strategy and avoid repeating mistakes and disappointment.

A comprehensive assessment considers a scar's location, depth, orientation, shape, contour, maturity, presence of hypertrophy or contracture, surface quality of the healed skin, pigmentation, and vascularity. Patient age and ethnicity also provide valuable information. All of these variables influence the surgical approach and prognosis.

Location

The location of a scar can affect its evolution after injury and treatment. Facial burn scars have a propensity to heal better than those found elsewhere on the body. Scars that align closely with RSTLs can blend in so well with adjacent skin that they appear like normal skin lines. The complexity of facial features requires an understanding of facial aesthetics. Tension must be eliminated in order to restore normal facial expression.

Nonfacial skin possesses a higher tension that typically causes scars to widen. This is especially true for the parasternal area, the deltoid-acromial-scapula region of the shoulder, and around the knee, frequently resulting in hypertrophy. In some areas of the body, especially the trunk, scar alignment with RSTLs does not tend

Table 1 Burn scar classification	
Mature scar	A flat, pale scar.
Immature scar	An erythematous, somewhat elevated scar that can be pruritic or painful. It is in the transitory process of remodeling.
Linear hypertrophic scar	An erythematous, elevated linear scar that is occasionally pruritic.
Diffuse hypertrophic scar	An erythematous, elevated wide-based scar that is occasionally pruritic and remains within the boundaries of the burn injury.

Adapted from Mustoe TA, Cooter RD, Gold MH, Hobbs FD, Ramelet AA, Shakespeare PG, Stella M, Téot L, Wood FM, Ziegler UE; International Advisory Panel on Scar Management. International clinical recommendations on scar management. Plast Reconstr Surg. 2002 Aug;110(2):560-71.

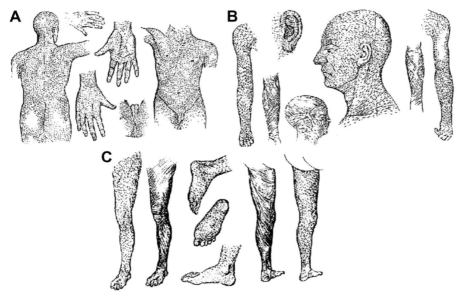

Fig. 6. (*A–C*) Langer's lines. (*From* On the anatomy and physiology of the skin. I. The cleavability of the cutis. (Translated from Langer, K. (1861). Zur Anatomie und Physiologie der Haut. I. Uber die Spaltbarkeit der Cutis. Sitzungsbericht der Mathematisch-naturwissenschaftlichen Classe der Kaiserlichen Academie der Wissenschaften, 44, 19.). Br J Plast Surg. 1978 Jan;31(1):3–8.)

to mitigate scar widening as much as is seen in the head and neck.[28,29]

Depth

The thickness of a mature burn scar is often variable because many burn scars, especially those that are diffuse, are heterogenous. Burn scars

can be incredibly thick, measuring more than 2 cm, or shallow, as is demonstrated in **Figs 8–10**.

Orientation

As discussed previously, the more closely a scar aligns with RSTLs, especially linear scars, the less tension is imposed on the scar and the more

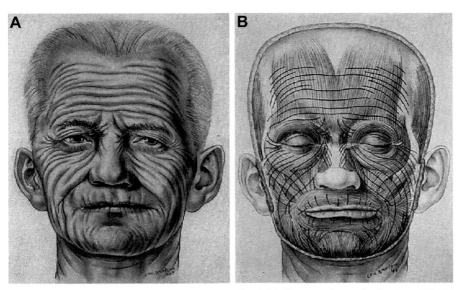

Fig. 7. (*A*) Relaxed skin tension lines (RSTLs) follow natural wrinkle lines, as shown in the face. (*B*) RSTLs are typically oriented perpendicular to the direction of the underlying muscles. (*From* Kraissl CJ. The selection of appropriate lines for elective surgical incisions. Plast Reconstr Surg (1946). 1951 Jul;8(1):1–28.)

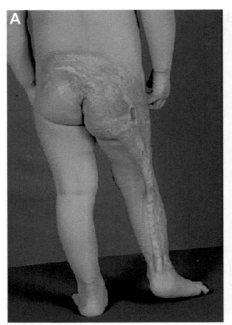
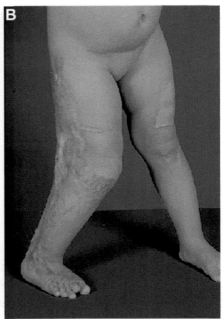

Fig. 8. (*A, B*) Young female patient with massive thick burn scars and contractures on the right leg. Note the downward displacement of the right buttock. The patient was unable to place her right heal on the ground and extend her knee normally.

likely it will not widen. Scars that are misaligned with RSTLs (along so-called antitension lines, or ATLs) can be made more aesthetically and functionally acceptable through local tissue rearrangement that reduces the tension.

Shape

Burn scars are very different from scars that are the result of sharp lacerations into or through the dermis. They tend to be primarily linear, primarily

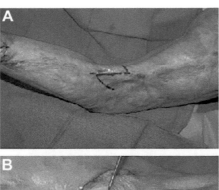
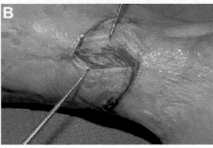
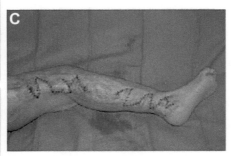

Fig. 9. (*A–C*) Thickened contractures along the lateral aspect of the leg and the popliteal fossa were released with multiple Z-plasties.

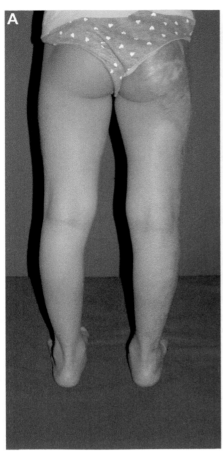
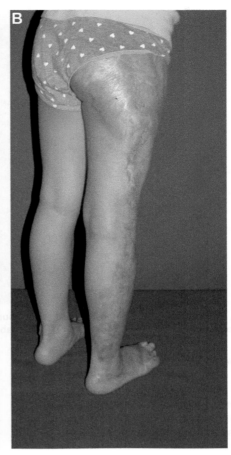

Fig. 10. (*A*, *B*) Four years after her first Z-plasty, the patient had a normal range of motion in her right knee and she was able to place her ankle on the ground. The scar's appearance and tension improved significantly. Her buttock was restored to a normal position.

diffuse, or a mixed combination of both. Both types can be improved by local tissue rearrangement (**Figs. 11–13**, Video 1). Narrow or linear scars tend to be more easily amenable to revision as the orientation of these scars is usually obvious. Curved scars can result in a raised deformity within the border of the scar. This phenomenon is caused by the trap door effect of contractile forces along the scar's margin acting like a purse string. Curvilinear and circumferential scars can be revised using multiple Z-plasties. Scar lengthening can be achieved by aligning the limbs of the Z-plasties with RSTLs to get the best possible outcomes. Diffuse areas of scarring, including hypertrophic scars, intervening areas of superficial scarring, and areas of normal skin, can be revised by finding focal areas within the diffuse scars that are suitable for Z-plasties (**Fig. 14**, Video 2). When large burn scars are predominantly linear, such as on the extremities, there are usually wide areas of scarring with severe hypertrophy that are

separated by narrower isthmuses of scar. The cumulative tension along the entire length is what creates the severe hypertrophy. This severe tension can often be almost completely eliminated by performing Z-plasties in the narrow areas of the scar alone. Laser treatment with LADD, time, and subsequent additional Z-plasties are all that is needed to correct the deformities.

Contour

The contour of scars that form after burn injury is often a mosaic of elevated and depressed tissue. The surface of a scar refers to the finer irregularities in the tissue's texture (relief).[30] Remodeling during wound healing involves a delicate and dynamic balance between the synthesis and degradation of extracellular matrix proteins. Disregulated inflammatory, proliferative, and remodeling phases of burn wounds can cause hypertrophic scars. They are a fibroproliferative disorder of the reticular

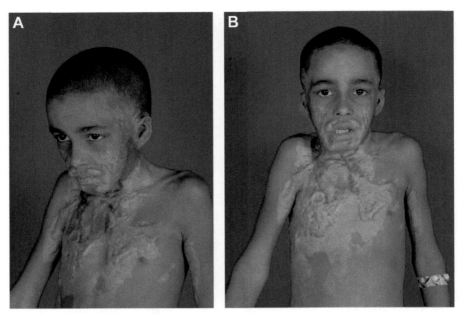

Fig. 11. (A, B) Young male with extensive third degree burns with diffuse scarring and a severe linear contracture with a chronic ulcer in the right axilla. Right shoulder abduction was limited to 30°.

dermis layer in which persistent inflammation and excessive angiogenesis and collagen production dominate. Hypertrophic scars are elevated, firm, and erythematous tissue that remains within the borders of the original wound. After the inciting burn injury, these scars evolve and mature over a period of 6 months to several years and respond predictably to their local environment as has already been discussed.[31]

The clinical features and progression of burn scars help one characterize hypertrophic scars. For a hypertrophic scar, it is essential to

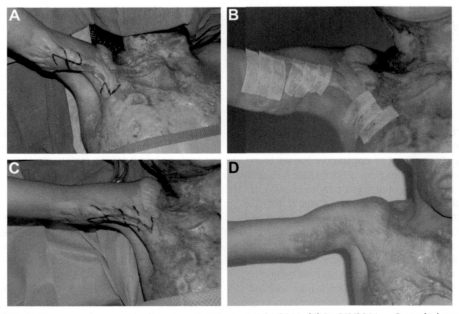

Fig. 12. (A) Z-plasties were done on the linear contracture on 1/24/2011. (B) By 2/9/2011, ~2 weeks later, the ulcer had healed. (C) Serial Z-plasties were carried out on 9/12/2011. (D). By 3/24/2014, the contracture had been eliminated.

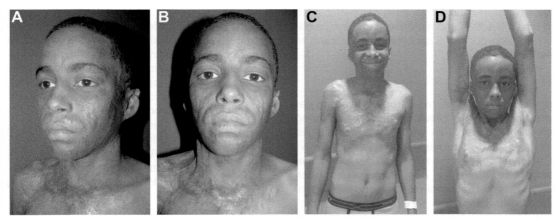

Fig. 13. (*A–D*) Three years after the first Z-plasties and 5 CO2 ablative fractional laser treatments, the appearance, elasticity, and sensation of the rehabilitated scars approximates normal.

understand factors that can influence how it presents. Is the scar misaligned and crossing RSTLs? Is it contracted and under tension? Does it involve a joint whose motion affects the tension on the scar?[32]

Depressed scars can result from tissue loss, fat atrophy, or adhesions that develop after burn injury. They are commonly the result of linear tension across a convex surface and can often be improved or eliminated by relieving the tension by lengthening the scars through local tissue rearrangement. Hypertrophic scars treated with excessive steroid injections can also become atrophic. Fat grafting and local tissue flaps can provide replacement volume to many depressed scars.[28,32]

This chapter focuses on the application of local tisuse rearrangement to hypertrophic scars, not keloids, which require a different approach to management. Keloids are a completely different fibroproliferative disorder that is like a benign tumor and are most often seen in genetically predisposed and dark-skinned individuals.[28,31–35]

Maturity

As previously mentioned, burn scars mature at different rates, depending on the type and age of a scar and the local, systemic, genetic, and lifestyle risk factors at play.[35] Scar analysis must consider a scar's age in the context of these other factors, as there is variability in scar presentation and prognosis.

The sooner scar analysis can be performed after burn injury, the earlier a scar diagnosis can be made and a treatment plan can be executed. Mitigating tension on an immature scar with compression or silicone dressings can obviate the need for surgical revision when the scar has matured. Similarly, a firm, erythematous hypertrophic scar that is

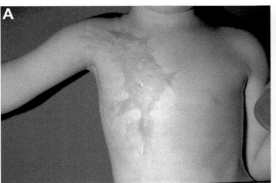
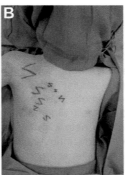
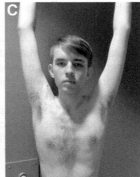

Fig. 14. (*A–C*) Young male with diffuse hypertrophic burn scars and contractures on the right chest. After undergoing Z-plasties within the scar tissue and ablative fractional CO2 laser treatments, full range of motion was restored and the scar's appearance was near normal.

only several months old in a fair-skinned patient will typically soften and flatten as it matures, motivating a non-operative conservative approach to treatment.[32]

Hypertrophy vs Contracture

As discussed above, hypertrophic scarring results from a fibroproliferative disorder involving persistent inflammation and excessive collagen synthesis.[31,33,34] Normal wound healing, however, involves contraction and when it is excessive, contractures develop. This phenomenon often occurs in areas of chronic tension and relaxation, such as the joints and perioral areas. Contractures can limit a joint's range of motion and impair function and quality of life.[36] Contractures can be diffuse or linear. A diffuse burn contracture often consists of a mixture of a large area of scarred skin with identifiable linear areas of scar within it that are amenable to local tissue rearrangement. This can decrease tension in the larger area (Fig. 14, Video 2). Linear contractures are a relatively narrow band of scar with elastic skin or scar on one or both sides making it an easy target for local tissue rearrangement of the surgeon's choosing.[36]

Pigmentation

Burn scars and contractures can have the same pigmentation as normal skin or they can be hypopigmented, hyperpigmented, or a combination of the two. Unfortunately, there are limited available effective treatments for dyschromia other than makeup. Local tissue rearrangement can revise a scar and help camouflage pigmentary abnormalities by using adjacent skin that has normal pigmentation. Kurup and colleagues recently reported improved pigmentation after treating hyperpigmented hypertrophic scars with laser-assisted drug delivery using an ablative fractional CO_2 laser.[37]

Vascularity

Vascularity and scar maturation are closely linked. The metabolic needs of a healing wound spur the formation of a growing microvascular network. As a scar matures and metabolic demands diminish, so too does the capillary bed. Marked erythema and increased vascularity help identify a scar as immature, prompting early intervention that lowers the likelihood of excessive scarring.[38]

Patient Age, Gender, Ethnicity, and Genetics

Remodeling and regeneration are integral to scar pathophysiology. It is well known to clinicians who regularly assess wounds and scars that aged skin heals and forms scars quite differently than does younger skin. As one ages, senescent cells accumulate, promoting persistent inflammation that causes a delay in wound healing and an impaired capacity for regeneration. Ultimately, this results in less scarring. This phenomenon is not entirely understood.[39–41]

Female gender, younger age (≤ 30 years), darker pigmented skin (Fitzpatrick skin type IV-VI), and people of African and Asian descent have been identified as risk factors for hypertrophic scarring and keloid formation following burn injury.[42–44]

THE DECISION TO REVISE A SCAR

The decision to surgically improve a scar depends on the scar's impact on function and aesthetics, a patient's goals, and what can realistically be achieved with reconstruction. The optimal treatment for scars is sometimes obvious. A linear facial burn scar that is hypertrophied and oriented against RSTLs can most likely be markedly improved with surgical revision and laser-induced rehabilitation. But in many cases identifying the key issues requires a more comprehensive assessment. A patient and the evaluating surgeon may judge functional and cosmetic impairment quite differently. A deformity that appears fairly inconsequential to the surgeon may cause a patient significant consternation. Similarly, functional deficits that are subtle to the observer may be substantial for the patient. Typically, a patient wants a scar totally removed, leaving the skin completely normal and unblemished when this is undoubtedly not feasible. Of course, this fact should be clearly communicated to the patient. It is critical for the surgeon to ascertain the differences in perspective and reach a consensus with the patient on the treatment plan and reasonable expectations for the intended outcome.[29] This approach ensures a greater likelihood of a successful result.

GOALS OF SCAR REVISION

The primary goal of scar revision is to improve a scar's appearance and make it less visible.[28,32] However, in cases in which a contracture limits function, contracture release is more important than addressing aesthetic concerns.

Any surgical technique employed in scar reconstruction should aim to: 1) decrease or eliminate tension by orienting a scar with RSTLs as closely as possible; 2) divide the scar into smaller components; and 3) level the surface of the scar to match adjacent normal skin. One should also minimize or eliminate any risk of iatrogenic injury or deformity associated with scar revision. Facial burn scars are unique given the visibility of the face and the potential impact deformities can have on alimentation, breathing, communication, and emotional expression. A patient's identity, emotional well-being, social engagement, and productivity are often at stake. To address facial deformities, a tension-free appearance that re-establishes the features, proportions, and expression of the face are the key objectives of reconstruction.[28,32] (**Fig. 15**).

Different surgical techniques have their indications and contraindications. They achieve each of the aforementioned aims to varying degrees, thus it is imperative to take the long view and carefully select the technique that can ultimately meet the needs of the patient and attain an optimal outcome.[28]

TIMING

The timing of local tissue rearrangement in scar revision falls into three phases: acute, intermediate, and late. In general, any reconstruction should be delayed until wounds have closed and inflammation has diminished. Local tissue rearrangement during this acute period has a limited indication and should be focused on closing wounds, eliminating exposure of vital structures, and preventing or treating scars and contractures that cause significant functional deficits.[36] Cases that warrant early intervention include eyelid ectropion, severe microstomia, fourth degree burn injuries necessitating flap coverage, and cervical contractures impairing breathing.[45]

The intermediate phase, during which time a burn scar is maturing, begins several months after injury and typically lasts for years. During this period, if tension on a scar is present, tension-relieving scar surgery is indicated and can improve the scar's appearance and elasticity. Local tissue operations can be utilized along with other noninvasive treatments, such as pressure therapy, silicone gels, splinting, and judicious steroid injections, as well as laser therapy.[36] Hypertrophic burn scars that are not under tension will usually improve given sufficient time. Revision of an erythematous, immature scar can be more challenging technically and can potentially aggravate the maturation process, leading to a less favorable outcome.[36]

The late phase occurs years after the initial trauma when deformities are fully mature and stable. Local scar tissue rearrangement is always appropriate in this stage when the deformity can be improved by using this technique.

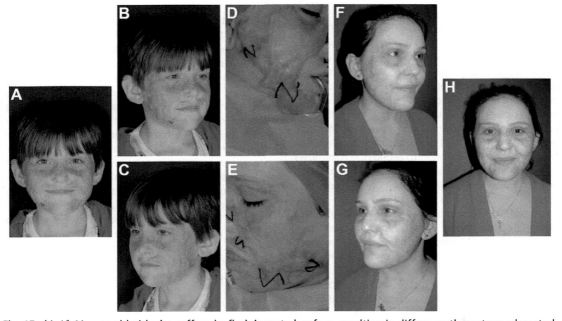

Fig. 15. (*A–H*) 11-year-old girl who suffered a flash burn to her face, resulting in diffuse erythematous, ulcerated, hypertrophic scars. Over a 7-year period, she underwent 4 Z-plasty procedures, 9 treatments with pulsed dye laser, and 10 treatments with a CO2 ablative fractional laser. No scars were ever excised, only dyspigmentation remained. Her face has a much more normal appearance and expression.

PRINCIPLES AND FUNDAMENTALS OF Z-PLASTY

The Z-plasty is the workhorse of local scar rearrangement. Before it was commonly known as a Z-plasty, the technique was first reported by W.E. Horner in 1837, who reconstructed a lower eyelid ectropion.[46,47] Since that time, numerous variations of the technique have been described but they are all based on the same underlying concept. The fundamentals of the Z-plasty, its fascinating history, and multiple variations are discussed in detail in many papers and textbooks.[48–57] Our focus here is limited to the use of the Z-plasty technique in local tissue rearrangement among burn patients (**Figs. 11–13**, Video 1).

A Z-plasty lengthens a scar and reduces its transverse dimensions by incising, elevating, and transposing across the scar's axis two opposing triangular flaps composed of scar tissue and normal or near normal tissue. This rearrangement reduces tension along the central line of the scar by recruiting a relative excess of lateral elastic tissue, lengthening the scar and inducing tissue remodeling that can lead to a thinner, softer, and more elastic scar. In addition, the technique makes the border of the scar irregular, enhancing camouflage.[48] It is of paramount importance that there is sufficient elasticity in the tissue adjacent to the scar so that the flaps can be properly mobilized. Meticulous technique is critical to achieving a successful outcome as flaps created with a Z-plasty are composed of scarred tissue. Flap tip necrosis can be avoided by making incisions perpendicular to the surface, ensuring that deeper tissue is included in the flap.[29] It is desirable to have the flaps look as much like cheesecake as possible. If the flaps look like apple pie with a crust and everything below it falling away, they will result in a dead space under the tip of the flap. This can lead to hematoma and ischemia, which can cause flap tip necrosis. Attention to technique minimizes this problem and enables the Z-plasty to be a powerful tool in dealing with contractures and scar irregularities in all types of tissues.

Z-plasties are typically described as dealing best with linear scars. Wide scars, however, can be very effectively narrowed by Z-plasty revision. A 60° Z-plasty lengthens a scar by 75% while narrowing it by approximately 30% (**Fig. 16**).[15] It is essential to note that skin tension, flap thickness, location, and other individual factors can alter the theoretic changes in length and width of a Z-plasty.[16] Because the shortest distance between two points is a straight line, as the lateral flaps are transposed with their base in normal tissue, a leveling effect is accomplished by the now transverse limb. This ability of a Z-plasty to elevate the surface of a depressed scar and lower the height of a hypertrophic scar, all without removing any scar or normal tissue, is one of its most powerful attributes.[50] These effects are noticeable immediately after the surgery is carried out.

In order for a Z-plasty to successfully lengthen and flatten a hypertrophic, contracted scar, the lateral limbs must go beyond the margin of the scar tissue. That fact determines the length of the central limb. The angles of the Z-plasty limbs do not need to be equal. They should be what is required for each scar deformity. Because Z-plasties are being performed in and on a mixture of scarred and unscarred tissue, the lateral limb lengths often need to be appropriately unequal. A scarred tissue flap is less elastic than a normal tissue one, requiring a longer length flap on the scarred side than the side with more normal tissue. All of these little soft tissue maneuvers make a big difference in the success or failure of the rearrangement operation.

Multiple Z-plasties can be used in an interrupted or contiguous fashion for long scars. Multiple smaller Z-plasties are very effective and are less noticeable than large Z-plasties with their conspicuous Z shape. When serial Z-plasties are incised, the flaps become 3-sided rhombic flaps and not 2-sided triangles.[49] The seemingly redundant tissue that results should not be trimmed but can be set into the opposing defect that is always present on the opposite side as the central limb is lengthened. This adds extra skin to the previously tightest line of the scar.

The 5-flap Z-plasty, aka the jumping man Z-plasty, consists of double opposing Z-plasties, with the resulting central V-shaped "5th flap" being advanced into a Y-shaped extension. This technique is useful most commonly when the scar that is being revised is a narrow, linear burn scar or a scar crossing a concavity such as the first web space, an axillary contracture, or a neck contracture. The 5-flap Z-plasty can be helpful to flatten dog ears and make for a more aesthetic closure. The 5th flap is a direct advancement flap so there must be tissue laxity at its base for there to be any significant additional releasing effect but it can often fit perfectly into the goals of the local tissue rearrangement.

OTHER LOCAL PLASTIC SURGERY TECHNIQUES

In addition to the Z-plasty, numerous other scar revision techniques have been developed to

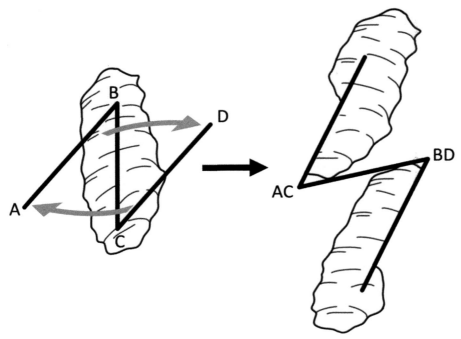

Fig. 16. Z-plasty. Three equal limbs and 60-degree angles theoretically increase a scar's length of a scar by 75% and narrow its width by 30%.

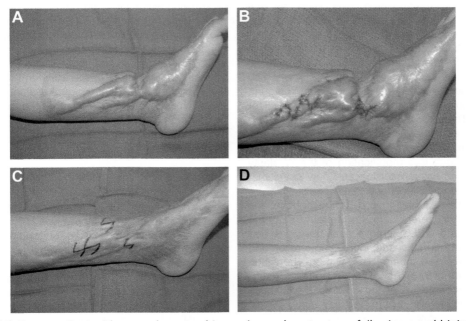

Fig. 17. (*A*) Young patient with severe hypertrophic scarring and contractures following a scald injury to the lower left leg and foot limiting range of motion in the ankle. (*B, C*) Z-plasties were done in 2012 and 2014. (*D*) Six years later, in 2018, the hypertrophic scarring had resolved and the patient's left leg and foot had a markedly improved appearance. Normal ankle function was restored.

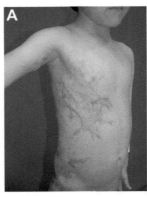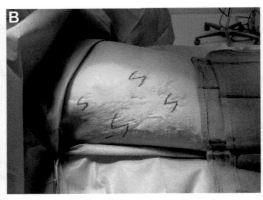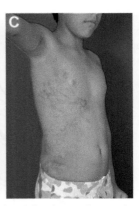

Fig. 18. (A–C) Young male with diffuse hypertrophic burn scars and contractures to the right chest. After undergoing Z-plasties within the scar tissue and CO2 ablative fractional laser treatments, full range of motion was restored and the scar's appearance was near normal.

make linear scars less noticeable. Two well-known techniques are the W-plasty and the geometric broken line closure (GBLC).

The W-plasty was introduced by Borges in 1959 and consists of the excision of an unfavorably oriented linear scar as well as a series of multiple small triangles of normal skin on either side. This creates an interdigitating and irregular closure but sacrifices adjacent normal skin in the process.[58]

Unlike the Z-plasty, the W-plasty does not lengthen a scar. Furthermore, it is an advancement flap, not a transposition flap such as the Z-plasty.[49] There are many iterations of the W-plasty reported in the literature.

The GBLC was first proposed by Webster in 1969.[59] This advancement flap technique is essentially a variation of the W-plasty whereby scar tissue is excised leaving the resulting wound with irregular edges that are brought together for closure. The opposing edges are composed of triangles, rectangles, squares, and semicircles formed in a random pattern that interdigitate. This technique is a modification of the W-plasty and requires tissue excision and new scars that have no camouflage effect.

Of the three techniques described above, the senior author prefers using the Z-plasty. Both the W-plasty and GBLC remove scar tissue as well as adjacent normal tissue, increasing tension and creating a fresh suture line without transition from abnormal to normal. There is no relief of tension or reorientation of the scarred area. These shortcomings are addressed by the classic Z-plasty. It maximally preserves normal tissue and facilitates the remodeling of the scar tissue over time by reducing tension (Figs. 8–10). The Z-plasty can decrease the height of hypertrophic

scars and elevate depressed scars by transposing flaps across the treated area from normal level to normal level and all without removing any normal tissue (Fig. 17).[50] A well-executed Z-plasty is often invisible to those unaware that the procedure was performed (see Fig. 14, see Video 2).[29] The current ability of Z-plasties to rehabilitate scar tissue has been enhanced by the synergistic benefits of laser therapy and topical medications. (Fig. 18, Videos 3–5).

As was previously discussed, the most important part of the art of local tissue rearrangement is knowing when it is appropriate, and recognizing when the nature and size of the burn scarring and deformity are too great to be reconstructed with local tissue alone. Fortunately, when that is the case, there are myriad local flaps, other techniques, and even free tissue transfer, that give us good options.[60,61] When careful evaluation of the deformities, however, reveals that the local tissue is adequate to achieve a satisfactory to excellent reconstruction, great benefit accrues to both the patient and the surgeon.

SUMMARY

Surgical revision of burn scars and contractures has improved greatly over the last 170 years. Advances in knowledge and understanding of burn pathophysiology, surgical anatomy, and surgical approaches have increased the number of options available to improve scars and treat associated deformities. Technological and pharmaceutical innovations have increased our ability to rehabilitate and utilize local scar tissue to achieve excellent results. Local tissue rearrangement was the surgical innovation that initiated that progress. Today it remains an enhanced, powerful, and minimally morbid reconstructive technique that should always be considered when treating burn patients and their deformities.

CLINICS CARE POINTS

> - The angles of Z-plasty limbs can be different. The lateral limb lengths are occasionally unequal.
> - Careful surgical technique makes a big difference in the success or failure of local tissue rearrangement operation.
> - Burn scar rehabilitation should eliminate tension and restore normal contours, features, and proportions as much as possible.
> - Laser therapy should be considered in any surgical plan for treating burn scars.
> - Scar excision should only be used in rare cases when other options are not available or suitable.

DISCLOSURE

The authors report no conflicts of interest or financial disclosures.

SUPPLEMENTARY DATA

Supplementary data related to this article can be found online at https://doi.org/10.1016/j.cps.2024.02.010.

REFERENCES

1. Robinson DH, Toledo AH. Historical development of modern anesthesia. J Invest Surg 2012;25(3):141–9.
2. Borges AF. Elective incisions and scar revision. Boston: Little Brown & Co. Inc; 1973.
3. McCurdy SL. Manual of orthopedic surgery. Pittsburgh, PA: Nicholson Press; 1898.
4. McCurdy SL. Z-plastic surgery: plastic operation to elongate cicatricial contraction of the neck, lips and eyelids and across joints. Surg Gynecol Obstet 1913;16:209–12.
5. Berger P. Autoplastie par dédoublement de la palmure et échange de lambeaux. Chirurgie ortopédique. Paris: Steinfeil. 1904:180-185.
6. Gillies H.D., Plastic surgery of the face based on selected cases of war injuries of the face including burns with original illustrations. H. Frowde; 1920.
7. Webster JP. The early history of the tubed pedicle flap. Surg Clin North Am 1959;39(2):261–75.
8. Davis JS. The relaxation of scar contractures by means of the Z-, or reversed Z-type incision: stressing the use of scar infiltrated tissues. Ann Surg 1931;94(5):871–84.
9. Asuku M, Yu TC, Yan Q, et al. Split-thickness skin graft donor-site morbidity: a systematic literature review. Burns 2021;47(7):1525–46.
10. Buta MR, Donelan MB. Evolution of burn care. Clin Plast Surg 2023;51(2):191–204.
11. Anderson RR, Parrish JA. Selective photothermolysis: precise microsurgery by selective absorption of pulsed radiation. Science 1983;220(4596):524–7.
12. Manstein D, Herron GS, Sink RK, et al. Fractional photothermolysis: a new concept for cutaneous remodeling using microscopic patterns of thermal injury. Lasers Surg Med 2004;34(5):426–38.
13. Alster TS. Improvement of erythematous and hypertrophic scars by the 585-nm flashlamp-pumped pulsed dye laser. Ann Plast Surg 1994;32(2):186–90.
14. Donelan MB, Parrett BM, Sheridan RL. Pulsed dye laser therapy and z-plasty for facial burn scars: the alternative to excision. Ann Plast Surg 2008;60(5):480–6.
15. Wenande E, Anderson RR, Haedersdal M. Fundamentals of fractional laser-assisted drug delivery: an in-depth guide to experimental methodology and data interpretation. Adv Drug Deliv Rev 2020;153:169–84.
16. Issler-Fisher AC, Waibel JS, Donelan MB. Laser modulation of hypertrophic scars: technique and practice. Clin Plast Surg 2017;44(4):757–66.
17. Choi KJ, Williams EA, Pham CH, et al. Fractional CO_2 laser treatment for burn scar improvement: a systematic review and meta-analysis. Burns 2021;47(2):259–69.
18. Klifto KM, Asif M, Hultman CS. Laser management of hypertrophic burn scars: a comprehensive review. Burns Trauma 2020;8:tkz002.
19. Miletta N, Siwy K, Hivnor C, et al. Fractional ablative laser therapy is an effective treatment for hypertrophic burn scars: a prospective study of objective and subjective outcomes. Ann Surg 2021;274(6):e574–80.
20. Mustoe TA, Cooter RD, Gold MH, et al. International clinical recommendations on scar management. Plast Reconstr Surg 2002;110(2):560–71.
21. Mustoe T.A., Chapter 9: International scar classification in 2019, In: Teot L., Mustoe T.A., Middlekoop E., et al., editors. Textbook on scar management: state of the art management and emerging technologies, 2020, Springer; Cham, 79–84.
22. Gibson T. Karl Langer (1819-1887) and his lines. Br J Plast Surg 1978;31(1):1–2.
23. Langer K. On the anatomy and physiology of the skin. I. The cleavability of the cutis. (Translated from

Langer, K. (1861). Zur Anatomie und Physiologie der Haut. I. Uber die Spaltbarkeit der Cutis. Sitzungsbericht der Mathematisch-naturwissenschaftlichen Classe der Kaiserlichen Academie der Wissenschaften, 44, 19. Br J Plast Surg 1978;31(1):3–8.

24. Carmichael SW. The tangled web of Langer's lines. Clin Anat 2014;27(2):162–8.

25. Borges AF, Alexander JE. Relaxed skin tension lines, Z-plasties on scars, and fusiform excision of lesions. Br J Plast Surg 1962;15:242–54.

26. Borges AF. Relaxed skin tension lines (RSTL) versus other skin lines. Plast Reconstr Surg 1984;73(1): 144–50.

27. Borges AF. Relaxed skin tension lines. Dermatol Clin 1989;7(1):169–77.

28. Borges AF. Scar analysis and objectives of revision procedures. Clin Plast Surg 1977;4(2): 223–37.

29. Donelan M.B., Surgical scar revision, In: Krakowski A.C. and Shumaker P.R., The Scar Book, 2017, Wolters Kluwer, chap 12, 170-194.

30. Powers M., Ozog D.M., Chaffins M.L. Scar Histopathology and Morphologic Classification. In: Krawkowski A.C., Shumaker P.R., eds. The Scar Book. Wolters Kluwer; 2017:chap 5.

31. Jeschke MG, Wood FM, Middelkoop E, et al. Nat Rev Dis Primers 2023;9(1):64.

32. Donelan M.B.. Facial Burn Treatment Principles. In: McCarthy J.G., Galiano R.D., Boutros S., eds. Current Therapy in Plastic Surgery. Elsevier; 2006:184-193.

33. Tredget EE, Levi B, Donelan MB. Biology and principles of scar management and burn reconstruction. Surg Clin North Am 2014;94(4): 793–815.

34. Finnerty CC, Jeschke MG, Branski LK, et al. Hypertrophic scarring: the greatest unmet challenge after burn injury. Lancet 2016;388(10052): 1427–36.

35. Ogawa R. The Most Current Algorithms for the Treatment and Prevention of Hypertrophic Scars and Keloids: A 2020 Update of the Algorithms Published 10 Years Ago. Plast Reconstr Surg 2022;149(1): 79e–94e.

36. Cartotto R, Cicuto BJ, Kiwanuka HN, et al. Common postburn deformities and their management. Surg Clin North Am 2014;94(4):817–37.

37. Kurup S, Travis TE, Shafy RAE, et al. Treatment of burn hypertrophic scar with fractional ablative laser-assisted drug delivery can decrease levels of hyperpigmentation. Lasers Surg Med 2023; 55(5):471–9.

38. Deng H, Li-Tsang CWP. Measurement of vascularity in the scar: a systematic review. Burns 2019;45(6): 1253–65.

39. Ding X, Kakanj P, Leptin M, et al. Regulation of the wound healing response during aging. J Invest Dermatol 2021;141(4S):1063–70.

40. Andrade AM, Sun M, Gasek NS, et al. Role of senescent cells in cutaneous wound healing. Biology 2022;11(12).

41. Colboc H., Meaume S., Scar and scarring in the elderly, In: Teot L., Mustoe T.A., Middlekoop E., et al., Textbook on scar management: state of the art management and emerging technologies, 2020, Springer, chap 44, 379-384.

42. Thompson CM, Hocking AM, Honari S, et al. Genetic risk factors for hypertrophic scar development. J Burn Care Res 2013;34(5):477–82.

43. Lawrence JW, Mason ST, Schomer K, et al. Epidemiology and impact of scarring after burn injury: a systematic review of the literature. J Burn Care Res 2012;33(1):136–46.

44. Nabai L, Pourghadiri A, Ghahary A. Hypertrophic scarring: current knowledge of predisposing factors, cellular and molecular mechanisms. J Burn Care Res 2020;41(1):48–56.

45. Donelan M.B., Liao E.C. Principles of Burn Reconstruction. In: Thorne C.H., ed. Grabb and Smith's Plastic Surgery. 7th ed. Lippincott Williams & Wilkins; 2014:142-154:chap 16.

46. Borges AF, Gibson T. The original Z-plasty. Br J Plast Surg 1973;26(3):237–46.

47. Horner W.E. Clinical Report on the Surgical Department of the Philadelphia Hospital, Blockley, for the months of May, June and July 1837. Am j Med Sci. 1837;21:105-106.

48. Hundeshagen G, Zapata-Sirvent R, Goverman J, Branski LK. Tissue Rearrangements: The Power of the Z-Plasty. Clin Plast Surg 2017;44(4): 805–12.

49. Shockley WW. Scar revision techniques: z-plasty, w-plasty, and geometric broken line closure. Facial Plast Surg Clin North Am 2011;19(3):455–63.

50. Marino H. Levelling of linear scars with Z-plasties. Clin Plast Surg Apr 1977;4(2):239–45.

51. Borges AF. Historical Review of Z-plastic Techniques. Clinics in Plastic Surgery 1977;4(2): 207–16.

52. Longacre JJ, Berry HK, Basom CR, Townsend SF. The effects of Z-plasty on hypertrophic scars. Scand J Plast Reconstr Surg 1976;10(2):113–28.

53. Borges A.F., The five single Z-plastics. Va Med Mon (1918). 1974;101(8):618-624.

54. Borges AF. The W-plastic versus the Z-plastic scar revision. Plast Reconstr Surg 1969;44(1):58–62.

55. McGregor IA. The z-plasty. Br J Plast Surg 1966; 19(1):82–7.

56. MCGREGOR IA. The theoretical basis of the Z-plasty. Br J Plast Surg 1957;9(4):256–9.

57. Rohrich RJ, Zbar RI. A simplified algorithm for the use of Z-plasty. Plast Reconstr Surg 1999;103(5): 1513–7.

58. Borges AF. Improvement of anti-tension line scars by the W-plastic operaiton. Br J Plast Surg 1959;12:29–33.

59. Webster RC. Cosmetic concepts in scar camouflaging - serial excisional and broken line techniques. Trans Am Acad Opthalmol Otolaryngol 1969;73(2):256–65.

60. Ogawa R. Usefulness of Local Flaps for Scar Contracture Release. In: Teot L., Mustoe T.A., Middlekoop E. Gauglitz G.G., eds. *Textbook on Scar Management: State of the Art Management and Emerging Technologies.* Springer; 2020:301-308:chap 35.

61. Ogawa R. Surgery for scar revision and reduction: from primary closure to flap surgery. Burns Trauma 2019;7:7.

Update on Hypertrophic Scar Management in Burn Patients

Rei Ogawa, MD, PhD, FACS

KEYWORDS

• Hypertrophic scar • Reticular dermis • Inflammation • Z-plasty • Local flap

KEY POINTS

- Hypertrophic scars arise due to persistent inflammation in the reticular dermis after burn injury.
- Several risk factors enhance the inflammation of hypertrophic scars, including local skin tension, estrogen, and hypertension.
- Conservative therapy should be used for prevention and before surgery is considered, including scar compression and fixation and local steroid administration.
- Steroid plaster effectively treats many hypertrophic scars.
- The most commonly used surgical methods for treating hypertrophic scars are Z-plasty, full-thickness skin grafting, and local flaps.

THE MECHANISMS THAT UNDERLIE HYPERTROPHIC SCAR FORMATION

To illustrate the mechanism by which hypertrophic scars arises, it is useful to compare burns to frostbite, which never develops into hypertrophic scars. While both damage the skin and produce seemingly similar ulcers, their wound-healing processes differ significantly. Thus, in burns, the heat causes the blood vessels to dilate and become permeable, which leads to immediate intense local inflammation. By contrast, in frostbite, the blood vessels constrict and sometimes freeze and rupture, causing the tissue to become ischemic. Eventually, the frostbitten area will demonstrate inflammation but because it arises only when the blood vessels have regenerated, this inflammation occurs well after the injury. These disparate responses are amplified in extensive burns and frostbite. Thus, extensive burns increase vascular permeability at a systemic level, which means there is an immediate need for significant fluid resuscitation. By contrast, in extensive frostbite, such large fluid requirements are rarely seen. These differences are also due to the respectively intense and absent initial inflammatory responses

that follow burn and frostbite. In burns, the intense inflammation prolongs the normally brief inflammatory stage of wound healing, and this can be worsened by repetitive stimuli (eg, local skin tension) that elevate vessel permeability. The resulting chronic inflammation then induces excessive blood vessel proliferation and fibroblast overproduction of collagen fibers, which respectively induce the redness and vertical growth of hypertrophic scars (the excessive collagen production explains why hypertrophic scars are categorized as a "dermal fibroproliferative disorder").[1] Indeed, hypertrophic scars are characterized histologically on the basis of collagen-fiber masses in the reticular dermis (dermal nodules), inflammatory cell infiltration, and neovascularization. These fundamental differences explain why burns, but not frostbite, are at extremely high risk of developing hypertrophic scars. Thus, targeting hypertrophic scar inflammation is the key to both prevention and treatment.[1]

While hypertrophic scar histology reveals changes in the reticular dermis (ie, nodules, inflammation, and neovascularization), the superficial papillary dermis and epidermis are relatively normal.[1] Moreover, first-degree or superficial

Department of Plastic, Reconstructive and Aesthetic Surgery, Nippon Medical School, Tokyo, Japan
E-mail address: r.ogawa@nms.ac.jp

Clin Plastic Surg 51 (2024) 349–354
https://doi.org/10.1016/j.cps.2024.02.001
0094-1298/24/© 2024 Elsevier Inc. All rights reserved.

dermal burns are less likely to result in hypertrophic scars (**Fig. 1**). Thus, hypertrophic scars generally only arise when the burn affects the deep dermis.

RISK FACTORS FOR HYPERTROPHIC SCAR FORMATION

Several risk factors promote chronic inflammation in burn wounds/scars and therefore hypertrophic scarring. One is tension on the skin at the burn site.[2] This factor arises in burns because the wound-healing process produces collagen fibers in the burn site, which hardens the tissue. When daily body movements pull on this hardened scar tissue, the force cannot be dissipated and inflammation is triggered. The mechanism underlying this response may relate to excessive mechanical stretching of the blood vessels in the scarred area, which increases vascular permeability. Indeed, studies have shown that stretching can enhance vascular permeability in even normal skin.[3]

An important systemic risk factor for hypertrophic scarring is female hormones. Recent research has shown that keloids, which are a more severe form of hypertrophic scars, can worsen during pregnancy.[4] Keloids also tend to be more prevalent in females.[5] These associations are likely to reflect high estrogen levels, which dilate blood vessels, thereby increasing local blood flow and intensifying peripheral tissue inflammation.

Hypertension is also considered to be a risk factor for worsening of hypertrophic scars. Studies show that hypertension associates with worse keloids and hypertrophic scars.[6]

These factors are useful for estimating the risk that a given burn will become a hypertrophic scar. Specifically, burns on areas that are prone to strong repetitive skin stretching (eg, the joints), burns in females or pregnant women, and burns in hypertensive patients all have a higher likelihood of developing into hypertrophic scars. This information can thus be used to institute early prevention measures.

PREVENTION OF HYPERTROPHIC SCARS

To prevent hypertrophic scars, it is essential to quickly resolve the inflammation in the burn wound. Practical methods to alleviate inflammation include (1) rest and immobilization of the wound, (2) compression of the wound, and (3) local administration of corticosteroids.[7]

Resting and immobilizing the wound is particularly crucial because continuously moving an inflamed burned/scarred area will exacerbate its inflammation. In fact, if the inflammation spreads to the surrounding healthy skin, the wound could develop into keloid. Methods to immobilize the wound include using bandages, supporters, corsets, knee braces, silicone gel sheets,[8] silicone tape, and adhesive tape.

Compressing the wound contracts the blood vessels, which reduces local inflammation. The best results occur when compression is sustained. Silicone gel sheets or sponges that are secured with bandages are suitable for this purpose. Pressure garments can also be used, although they may be uncomfortable when the weather is hot and humid.

Local corticosteroid can be administered with tape preparations. In particular, deprodone propionate $20\mu g/cm2$ plaster (Eclar plaster) reduces local inflammation very effectively[9,10] (**Figs. 2 and 3**). Compared to halogenated steroids such as fludroxicortide (the tape that delivers this steroid is Drenison tape), deprodone propionate is non-halogenated and therefore has fewer side effects such as capillary dilation. This makes Eclar plaster easier to use. When using Eclar plaster, it is important to cut it so that it is slightly larger than the scar area; this will prevent the inflammation from spreading to the surrounding skin. Given that the concentration of the medication decreases over 24 hours, it is recommended to

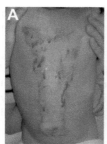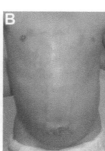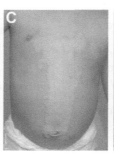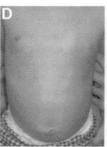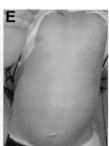

Fig. 1. Typical course of wound healing after a superficial dermal burn. (*A*) Immediately after burn injury. (*B*) Two weeks, (*C*) 4 weeks, (*D*) 6 weeks, and (*E*) 2 months after injury. Generally, if the injury does not reach the reticular dermis, the wound-healing course will progress smoothly and wound/scar inflammation will subside quickly.

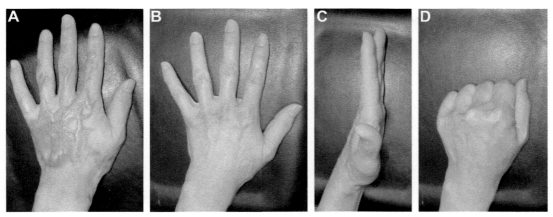

Fig. 2. Deprodone propionate plaster treatment of a burn-induced hypertrophic scar on the dorsum of the left hand of a woman in her 40s. (*A*) Before treatment 1 year after the burn injury was sustained. (*B–D*) Three years after starting treatment. The only treatment provided was Eclar plaster. The scar improved without any contractures.

replace it at least once a day. It is good practice to gently remove it during bathing, wash the scarred area, and apply a new piece after bathing.

Injections of triamcinolone acetonide (Kenacort) can also be considered, but being a halogenated steroid, it is prone to causing capillary dilation. Consequently, its use should be minimized.

CONSERVATIVE TREATMENT OF HYPERTROPHIC SCARS

In Japan, steroid plaster is the first-line therapy once hypertrophic scars form.[9] Thus, when a

burn wound becomes red and raised, which signifies hypertrophic scar formation, the first treatment is daily corticosteroid tape (Eclar plaster) application. If there is epidermal erosion or it arises during plaster administration, ointment should be applied to the eroded part and Eclar plaster should be placed around it. It should be noted that untreated hypertrophic scarring generally peaks at 3 to 6 months before gradually subsiding, unless there are systemic or local risk factors; in this case, the scar can take more than 5 years to mature. Using Eclar plaster can shorten this period but because it takes time to achieve the desired

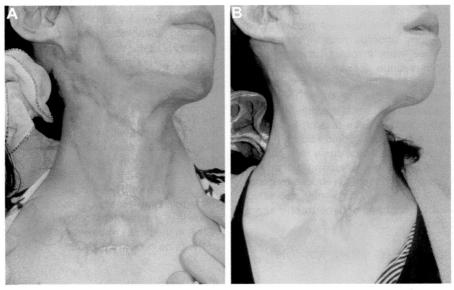

Fig. 3. Deprodone propionate plaster treatment of a burn-induced hypertrophic scar on the neck of a woman in her 30s. (*A*) Before treatment 6 months after the burn injury was sustained. (*B*) Eighteen months after starting treatment. The only treatment provided was Eclar plaster. The scar improved without any contractures.

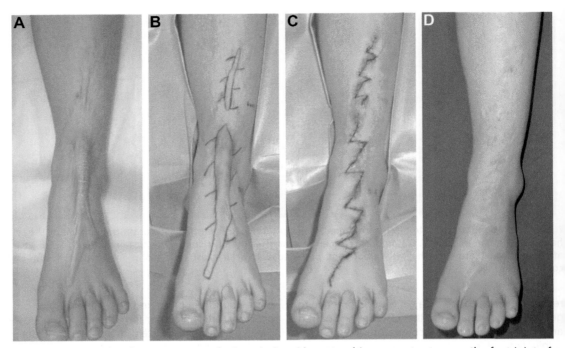

Fig. 4. Resection and Z-plasty treatment of a burn-induced hypertrophic-scar contracture on the foot joint of a pre-teen girl. (*A*) Before surgery. (*B*) Design of resection of as much of the hypertrophic scars as possible and the subsequent multiple Z-plasties. (*C*) Immediately after surgery. (*D*) Eighteen months after surgery. The resection and Z-plasties completely released the contracture. (*From:* Ogawa R. Surgery for scar revision and reduction: from primary closure to flap surgery. Burns Trauma. 2019 Mar 1;7:7)

outcomes, this should be explained to the patient in advance.

Even when using Eclar plaster, the inflammation sometimes does not subside. In this case, the case should be examined for the presence of factors that could incite local inflammation. For example, the patient has not kept the wound at rest because they undergo routine exercise at the gym or their work involves physical labor. Other examples include scratching due to itchiness, severe hypertension, or administration of female hormones. However, if these modifiable factors are absent, additional treatment should be considered alongside Eclar plaster.

For widespread hypertrophic scars where inflammation does not subside easily, oral corticosteroids may be tried. Generally, 5 mg/d of prednisone administered for 3 months reduces systemic inflammation. Anti-allergic drugs may also effectively relieve the symptoms of hypertrophic scars, including itching.

SURGICAL TREATMENT OF HYPERTROPHIC SCARS

If conservative treatments are not effective and the hypertrophic scar transitions to scar contracture, surgical treatment becomes an option.[11,12]

Z-plasty

Since skin tension prolongs inflammation, hypertrophic scars should be segmented.[12] Indeed, segmented scars mature faster than long linear scars. Zig-zag incision-and-suture strategies, including Z-plasty and W-plasty, are good for releasing linear scar contractures and tension. Z-plasty is better than W-plasty in terms of tension reduction. This means that W-plasty rather than Z-plasty is a good choice for facial hypertrophic scars.

Ideally, the triangular flaps of the Z-plasty should not include scarred skin. Therefore, if the width of the burn scar is within the range that can be sutured, it is advisable to completely excise the hypertrophic scar and perform a Z-plasty in the surrounding area (**Fig. 4**). This is because healthy skin extends readily after surgery, thereby effectively releasing tension, whereas scarred skin is much less extensible. Moreover, including scarred tissue in the flaps increases the risk that the edges of the flaps become necrotic.

Skin Graft

Split-thickness skin grafts (STSG) tend to develop severe secondary contractures and should

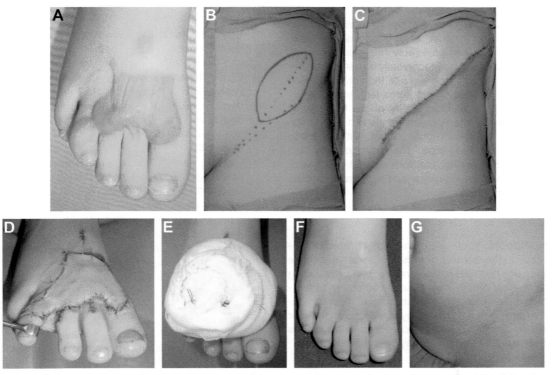

Fig. 5. Full-thickness skin grafting of a burn-induced hypertrophic scar on the foot dorsum of a child. (A) Before surgery. (B) Design of the skin graft on the donor site in the inguinal region. (C) After donor-site closure. (D) After applying the skin graft to the excised scar site. (E) Tie-over fixation. (F, G) View of the recipient (F) and donor site (G) 1 year after surgery. The graft healed without any significant issues. The color and texture of the graft were similar to that of the surrounding skin.

therefore be followed by secondary scar reconstruction with full-thickness skin grafts (FTSG), which are much less prone to such contractures (Fig. 5). However, FTSGs survive less well than STSGs because of the increased diffusion distance and the longer time that these grafts need before they achieve complete revascularization.

Local Flaps

Since skin grafts do not expand markedly, they tend to result in circular pathologic scars around the grafted skin. If these scars are on a major joint, they can generate secondary contractures. By contrast, local flaps expand naturally after surgery and thus are not prone to postsurgical contractures.

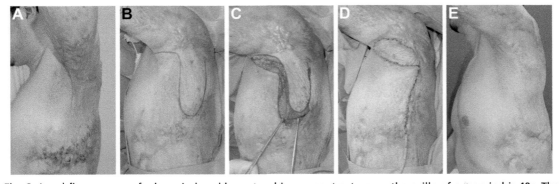

Fig. 6. Local-flap surgery of a burn-induced hypertrophic-scar contracture on the axilla of a man in his 40s. The flap was a transposition flap. (A) Before the operation. (B) Flap design. (C) Flap elevation. (D) Immediately after flap transfer. (E) One year after the operation. Although the flap contained scarred skin, the fact that the flap had a skin pedicle meant that it could expand after surgery. Recurrence of the hypertrophic scars was not observed.

Various local flaps are useful for releasing scar contractures caused by hypertrophic scars, including advancement, rotation, and transposition flaps. These flaps should preferably have skin pedicles because although it is technically easier to transfer island flaps to the recipient site than skin-pedicled flaps, they release contractures less effectively.[13] The postoperative extensibility of the flap should be considered when determining which flap design is optimal for the individual patient. With regard to the skin-pedicled flaps, the transposition flap (Fig. 6) and square flap methods are particularly useful for reconstructing major joint hypertrophic scars and scar contractures.

SUMMARY

Hypertrophic scars are caused by chronic inflammation in the reticular dermis. Consequently, these scars are best prevented and treated by reducing the tension on the wound/scar and using corticosteroid tape to alleviate inflammation. If corticosteroid tape does not prevent hypertrophic scarring or fails to improve existing scars and contractures arise, surgical treatment may be considered.

CLINICS CARE POINTS

- Hypertrophic scars after burns are persistent inflammation in scars or the dermis.
- The most important factor that exacerbates inflammation is tension.
- For treatments that directly reduce inflammation, corticosteroids are effective, especially in the form of tapes/plasters.
- Treatments to relieve tension include Z-plasty, thick skin grafting, and local flap surgery.

DISCLOSURE

There are no conflicts of interest.

REFERENCES

1. Ogawa R. Keloid and hypertrophic scars are the result of chronic inflammation in the reticular dermis. Int J Mol Sci 2017;18(3):606.
2. Ogawa R. Mechanobiology of scarring. Wound Repair Regen 2011;19(Suppl 1):s2–9.
3. Demir T, Takada H, Furuya K, et al. Role of skin stretch on local vascular permeability in murine and cell culture models. Plast Reconstr Surg Glob Open 2022;10(1):e4084.
4. Park TH, Chang CH. Keloid recurrence in pregnancy. Aesthetic Plast Surg 2012;36(5):1271–2.
5. Noishiki C, Hayasaka Y, Ogawa R. Sex differences in keloidogenesis: an analysis of 1659 keloid patients in Japan. Dermatol Ther 2019;9(4):747–54.
6. Arima J, Huang C, Rosner B, et al. Hypertension: a systemic key to understanding local keloid severity. Wound Repair Regen 2015;23(2):213–21.
7. Ogawa R. The most current algorithms for the treatment and prevention of hypertrophic scars and keloids: a 2020 update of the algorithms published 10 Years ago. Plast Reconstr Surg 2022;149(1):79e–94e.
8. O'Brien L, Jones DJ. Silicone gel sheeting for preventing and treating hypertrophic and keloid scars. Cochrane Database Syst Rev 2013;2013(9):CD003826.
9. Ogawa R, Akita S, Akaishi S, et al. Diagnosis and treatment of keloids and hypertrophic scars-Japan scar workshop consensus document 2018. Burns Trauma 2019;7:39.
10. Goutos I, Ogawa R. Steroid tape: a promising adjunct to scar management. Scars Burn Heal 2017;3. 2059513117690937.
11. Orgill DP, Ogawa R. Current methods of burn reconstruction. Plast Reconstr Surg 2013;131(5):827e–36e.
12. Ogawa R. Surgery for scar revision and reduction: from primary closure to flap surgery. Burns Trauma 2019;7:7.
13. Yoshino Y, Kubomura K, Ueda H, et al. Extension of flaps associated with burn scar reconstruction: a key difference between island and skin-pedicled flaps. Burns 2018;44(3):683–91.

Emerging Technologies

Sigrid A. Blome-Eberwein, MD

KEYWORDS

• Emerging technologies • Skin substitutes • Grafting techniques

KEY POINTS

- Recent and ongoing technological developments have had a large impact on burn care and wound management.
- Integration of artificial intelligence with clinical decision support tools has allowed for more accurate burn depth measurement and administration of supportive care.
- When treating full-thickness burns, there are a growing number of synthetic, biological, and hybrid alternatives/adjuncts to autologous split-thickness.
- Scar contractures can significantly decrease a patient's range of motion and degrade their quality of life, though newer, minimally invasive techniques to release contractures are proving effective.

INTRODUCTION

Burn care as a surgical specialty evolved in the 1970s when Zora Janzekovic introduced surgical eschar removal and early skin grafting.[1,2] Before that point, burn care focused on wound care instead of surgery. The early removal of eschar, earlier wound closure, and intensive care support for the patient led to significant improvements in survival and outcomes.[2] Emerging technologies are constantly helping to improve burn care even further. Diagnostic, intensive care, surgical, reconstruction techniques, and technological advances are being continuously developed, many of which will be discussed here. While far from an all-inclusive list, the technologies discussed have been chosen by the author as clinically relevant today and are divided into 3 areas: advances in acute burn care, wound closure, and reconstruction.

ACUTE BURN CARE

Objective Injury Depth Evaluation

Two factors determine burn severity: (1) burn size, or the extent of the injured skin surface area, measured in total burn surface area (in clinical practice, more commonly estimated by charts, computer programs, and applications) and (2) burn depth. The depth of a burn injury cannot be as easily determined as the size. Ultimately, a biopsy determines the actual depth of injury, but since most burn wounds contain several regions with variable injury depth, this method is not clinically relevant. Recent technologies in this area include optical devices like the laser Doppler imager, the Spectral MD camera, forward looking infrared (FLIR), and the indocyanine green dye technique, which all measure blood perfusion and hemoglobin reflection/absorption by the tissue (Figs. 1–4). Most recently, image interpretation has been augmented by deep learning algorithms.[3,4] Optical imaging is beneficial for measuring multiple properties of soft tissue.[5] Because of the wide variety of ways different soft tissues absorb and scatter light, optical imaging can measure metabolic changes that are early markers of abnormal functioning of organs and tissues.[5]

Fluid Resuscitation

After burn injury, fluid resuscitation that is both adequate and precisely individualized is essential to ensure survival, prevent organ dysfunction (kidney failure, compartment syndrome, cardiac failure, and so forth), and provide optimal skin perfusion to prevent burn wound progression. An artificial intelligence–supported resuscitation support

---

Department of Burn Surgery, University of South Florida Morsani College of Medicine, Lehigh Valley Health Network, 1200 S Cedar Crest Boulevard, Allentown, PA 18103, USA
E-mail address: sigri.blome-eberwein@lvhn.org

Clin Plastic Surg 51 (2024) 355–363
https://doi.org/10.1016/j.cps.2024.02.002
0094-1298/24/© 2024 Elsevier Inc. All rights reserved.

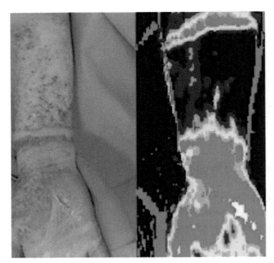

Fig. 1. Laser Doppler Imaging of a burn wound. Hop, M.J., Hiddingh, J., Stekelenburg, C.M. et al. Cost-effectiveness of laser Doppler imaging in burn care in the Netherlands. BMC Surg 13, 2 (2013). https://doi.org/10.1186/1471-2482-13-2.

system has been developed by ArcosTM. This system supports individualizing fluid administration through real-time feedback systems not dependent on human data entry and interpretation alone.[6]

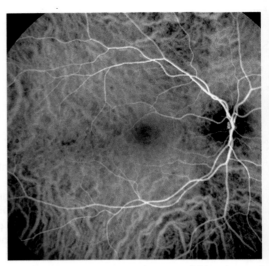

Fig. 3. Indocyanine green image of blood vessels (eye). This image was originally published in the Retina Image Bank® website. Gareth Lema MD, PhD. Photographer Sandra Boglione.Polypoidal Choroidal Vasculopathy - IVFA/ICGA. Retina Image Bank. 2018; 28352. © The American Society of Retina Specialists.

Pain Control

Adequate pain control is prominent in acute burn care, wound debridement, dressing changes, and daily personal hygiene. A nursing-driven nitrous oxide pain protocol, administered via the Pro-Nox device, has been developed and is supported by the American Association of Anesthesiologists and others.[7] Nitrous oxide provides pain relief by acting as a partial opioid receptor agonist. It does not get metabolized and is excreted by exhalation (**Fig. 5**). Using this technique for moderate sedation enables the providers and caretakers of a burn patient to provide adequate wound care without the excessive use of opioids, thereby decreasing the contribution to opioid dependency and abuse.[7]

Removal of Burn Eschar

Early and complete removal of burn eschar, which means necrotic tissue, contributes most significantly to survival and outcome. Throughout the years, since the introduction of surgical excision, the technique evolved from the excision down to fascia level to the modern tangential excision of only perceived necrotic tissue. Preservation of dermal elements and fat tissue, if possible, has shown to yield better long-term outcomes including function and esthetic appearance. Since the technology for real-time exact determination of burn depth remains to be developed, the decision of depth of excision presently depends on the

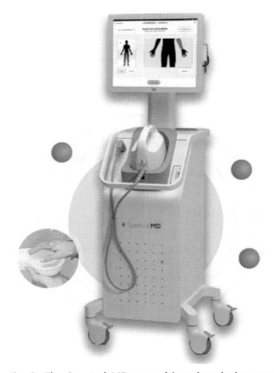

Fig. 2. The Spectral MD wound imaging device uses artificial intelligence and multispectral imaging to assess wound severity. Used with permission from Spectral AI, Inc.

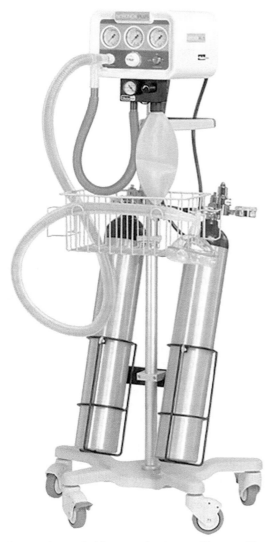

Fig. 4. Nitrous Oxide setup by Porter. Nitronox Plus, Porter Instrument, Hatfield, PA.

surgeon's experience. Because of the many contour variations and skin thickness differences in different parts of the human body, over-excision and under-excision are common. Clinical indicators like punctate bleeding and the color of the underlying tissue are notoriously imprecise. Recently, an enzyme has been introduced, based on bromelain, which appears to be powerful enough to enzymatically degrade necrotic tissue while preserving healthy tissue within a reasonable time frame.[8] After application and incubation of the enzyme, the necrotic tissue disintegrates enough to be removed by scraping (**Fig. 6**). The process is painful and requires significant pain control, and although significantly reduced when compared to surgical excision, a risk of bleeding remains.[8]

Other more precise technologies for eschar removal include the Versajet device, which works on the basis of hydro-dissection by the Venturi effect, cutting (indiscriminately) with a high-velocity stream of water, which creates "suction" at the same time. The Versajet device is most useful for softer tissue like granulation tissue. Removing hard burn eschar can be time consuming. The Misonix ultrasound device—which works on the principle of ultrasonic destruction of cell walls, combined with suction—is beneficial in contaminated wounds because it destroys bacterial cell walls some distance into tissue. (The Sonicare toothbrush works similarly, destroying bacterial cell walls in gum recesses, without destroying the mucosa). The Amalgatome is a device originally developed for meat processing. A rotating disk knife, set to a certain thickness, is used to "slice" through tissue. It can be used for burn eschar excision and is particularly helpful in concave body areas, fat tissue, and large surface areas like the back or chest. It leaves a smoother wound bed and cleaner edges than the Weck or Watson knife. In addition, it is now widely used for skin harvesting.[9]

WOUND CLOSURE

Deep burn wounds have little or no intrinsic healing potential because the epidermal stem cell layer was destroyed. Wound closure ultimately depends on autologous epidermal and dermal cells being introduced into the wound bed to achieve closure. Skin grafting, whether full-thickness or split-thickness, has been the standard of care. The creation of a significant donor site, with its sequelae and complications, is one major drawback of this technique, as well as significant scarring. Cultured cells were introduced in 1975 by Rheinwald and Green and have been used in extensive burn wounds since 1981.[10] A significant time delay of approximately 3 weeks is necessary to grow the cell grafts in a commercial laboratory, and the purely epidermal cell sheets need a dermal component to engraft. A more recent solution for point-of-care epidermal coverage was developed by Dr. Fiona Woods, using a small split-thickness skin donor to process cell suspension, which can be sprayed onto the prepared wound bed in a maximum 1:80 expansion ratio.[11] The preparation kit is commercially available in the United States as Recell by Avita Medical. Other applications of the autologous cell suspension include repigmentation in vitiligo, augmented donor site healing, and healing of traumatic wounds.

A self-assembled skin substitute consisting of fibroblasts and keratinocytes is currently under

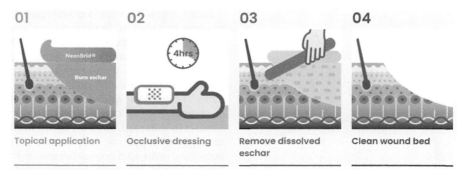

01 Topical application
02 4hrs Occlusive dressing
03 Remove dissolved eschar
04 Clean wound bed

Fig. 5. Enzymatic debridement process. Used with permission from MediWound.

investigation.[12] Many other tissue engineering projects are currently under investigation in animal and human trials, all based on a scaffold, whether synthetic or biological, which populates with fibroblasts and keratinocytes. In addition, researchers are investigating cell modulation and bioprinting.

The Meek technique is widely accepted globally to cover extensive burn wounds with split-thickness grafts.[13] Any small piece of split-thickness skin graft (STSG) is placed on a carrier after being cut into 0.4 × 0.4 cm squares. The carrier is folded in a plisse-type fashion, and the little squares of skin are separated by opening the plisse folds. The entire carrier with STSG is then placed on the wound, allowing from 1:2 to 1:8 expansion.[13]

Whether biological or synthetic, skin substitutes are an ever-expanding field of emerging technology; some are designed as epithelial cover substitutes, some as dermal, and some as both. Relevant in current burn care are several dermal substrates with a synthetic epidermal placeholder, some dermal scaffolds without cover, and epidermal substrates.[14] Integra, BTM, Biobrane (not available in the United States and mostly established for partial thickness wounds), Matriderm, Hyalomatrix, and Pelnac all function as (partially) biologic scaffolds for dermal regeneration with a temporary synthetic cover to mimic epidermal coverage until autologous epidermis can be transplanted (**Figs. 7** and **8**).[15] On the other hand, Primatrix, Supra SDRM, Matriderm, Acell, Alloderm, and fish skin function as dermal scaffolds, promoting the ingrowth of fibroblasts and the formation of granulation tissue for wound bed conditioning without a cover membrane.[15] These substances can sometimes bridge small areas of avascular structures like exposed tendons and bone and avoid chronic open wound formation in those areas. In addition, the scar contracture after dermal scaffold use is often decreased, thereby preventing some degree of joint contractures in the long term. Epidermal skin substitutes currently in use are cryopreserved or glycerol-preserved cadaver allodermis and xenografts like fish or porcine grafts, including all their processed/acellular derivatives (amniotic substrates, mucosal substrates, and so forth) which are biologic, as well as Suprathel and Biobrane, which are synthetic (**Fig. 9**).[15] These protect the wound's natural/intrinsic healing potential, preventing infection and augmenting cell proliferation. While Suprathel is biodegradable and does not integrate into the wound, Biobrane (including the cell-seeded derivatives Dermagraft, Apligraf, and so forth) needs to be removed and does integrate into the wound bed if the dermal injury extends beyond the papillary dermis.[14]

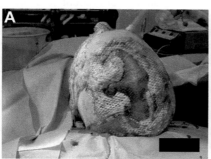
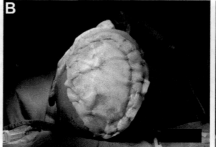
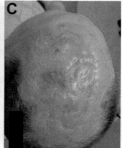

Fig. 6. BTM on exposed bone (skull): Injury, BTM in place, Skin graft healed on top of BTM after 12 weeks.

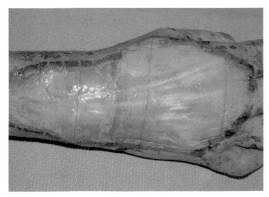

Fig. 7. Integra on exposed tendon, ready for skin grafting.

BURN RECONSTRUCTION

The prevalence of developing a hypertrophic scar following a burn-related injury has been reported to be as high as 70%. These scars can be cosmetically unappealing, with associated symptoms of pruritus, pain, and restricted range of motion, which can impair a person's quality of life. Such scars are thought to develop from patterns of dysregulation of normal wound healing after trauma to the skin. Surgical scar removal and contracture release remain important corrective therapies; however, these techniques have high risks of scar recurrence.[16] Nonsurgical interventions are often attempted prior to surgical interventions to inhibit or slow scar progression. Nonsurgical interventions include pressure garments, silicone gel sheeting, intralesional injections, cryotherapy, radiation therapy, and laser and light therapy. Laser and light therapies have now emerged as minimally invasive, low-risk therapies with a short postoperative recovery period.[17]

Prevention and release of contractures using skin substitutes/dermal templates play a significant role in modern burn reconstruction. All of the previously mentioned modalities have been used. The most recently developed substrates are BTM and Zurich skin. Most substrates require the release of contractures and application of

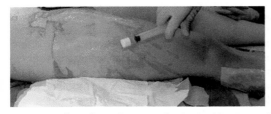

Fig. 8. Recell epidermal autograft suspension sprayed onto dermal wound bed.

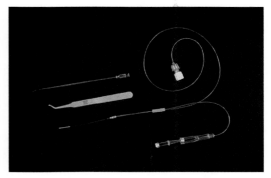

Fig. 9. Microdialysis catheter.

dermal substrate, followed by a period of ingrowth of fibroblasts and the formation of a dermislike layer that will then be skin grafted.[18] (See earlier description in acute burn treatment)

Flap reconstruction is a common technique in burn reconstruction. Newer preoperative mapping techniques for supplying vessels and postoperative monitoring devices have been developed.[19] Thermography (FLIR) is based on heat detection and is used to map vessels preoperatively. Similarly, indocyanine green fluoroscopy can be used to map blood vessels preoperatively and postoperatively. Laser Doppler flowmetry is based on the reflection of laser light by erythrocytes. Microlight-guided spectrophotometry uses optical techniques to distinguish well perfused and not well-perfused tissues. The amount of light absorption by hemoglobin depends on its oxygenation level and the wavelength of the light. By analyzing the spectrum of the reflected light, the device can calculate the tissue's oxygen saturation and blood flow. Tissue pH monitoring and microdialysis are 2 other invasive monitoring techniques based on the chemical composition of interstitial fluid in the tissues (Fig. 10). Technetium-99 m sestamibi scintigraphy and perfusion-weighted MRI are 2 of the less studied and more expensive modalities.[19,20]

Fat grafting has been used in burn reconstruction, mainly to improve contour irregularities and to treat skin-to-muscle or tendon adhesions (Fig. 11). Modern harvesting techniques (laser or ultrasound-assisted) can be used; however, manual harvesting usually yields sufficient material (Fig. 12).[21]

Botulinum toxin is used in burn reconstruction to augment contracture release procedures by relaxing the contracted underlying musculature. It is also believed that the relaxation of myofibroblasts is an adjunct in keloid and hypertrophic scar treatment.[22] There is emerging evidence that it can influence fibroblast activity and minimize tension around the scar by muscular chemo-immobilization.[23]

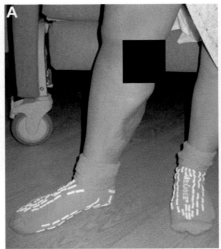
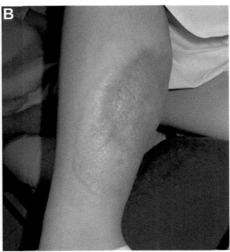

Fig. 10. Adherent scar before and after fat grafting.

Using self-inflating hydrophilic expanders has dramatically simplified tissue expansion for burn reconstruction, especially in children (**Fig. 13**).[24,25] Unfortunately, these devices are only approved in mini-formats for ear, nose, and throat doctors and dentistry in the United States.

Transplantation science and practice advances have made hand/face and abdominal wall transplantation possible.[26] According to a recent publication on face transplant outcomes, there have been 48 face transplantations worldwide in 46 patients since the first report of this procedure in 2005. Eleven of those recipients were burn survivors. Nine of 46 patients have since died and 2 transplants have been reported as rejected. The long-term recovery of facial expression was measured in the aforementioned study as restoration of facial motor function and smile at roughly 40%. A better outcome (42.7%) was found when

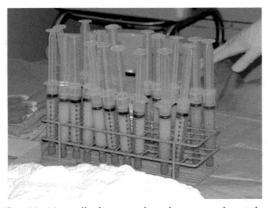

Fig. 11. Manually harvested and processed autologous fat used for scar fat grafting.

nerve coaptation was performed at the distal branch level.[27–29] The long-term need for immunosuppression and psychological issues in the transplantation of non-vital organs limit its implementation in burn reconstruction in most burn survivors. Immunologic risk factors also need to be taken into account when undertaking face transplantation because patients with a past medical history of burns and transfusions may have developed immunosensitization.[28]

Minimally invasive techniques are understandably popular in the burn survivor community. Subcutaneous contracture band release, microneedling, and laser/light-based therapies have gained wide acceptance recently.

Fractional laser therapies have made scar treatment with ablation carbon dioxide (CO_2) lasers feasible. Burn scars resulting from deep dermal or full-thickness injuries have a relatively normal epidermis on a very abnormal dermis, which usually does not contain dermal adnexa and, therefore, no stem cell nests of epidermal cells. Treating a burn scar with ablation, be it by thin excision, dermabrasion, or ablation laser, would cause an open wound that resembles a new full-thickness burn, requiring epidermal coverage for healing. Fractional and nonablative lasers can selectively injure the abnormal scar and stimulate remodeling without significant epidermal injury.[17] Fractional lasers, such as fractional CO_2 and fractional erbium: YAG lasers, create controlled micro-injuries within the scar tissue.[30] This stimulates collagen remodeling and tissue regeneration, leading to a smoother, more flexible scar. Laser therapy can also reduce scar redness and improve skin texture, helping patients regain confidence and function.[30,31]

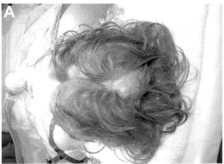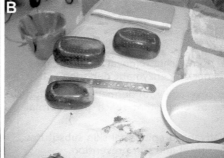

Fig. 12. Self-inflated expanders in situ and removed.

Subcutaneous contracture band release can be performed under local anesthesia. Subcutaneous bands of scar tissue, often restricting the range of motion and leaving the burn survivor with the feeling of tightness, can be released by passing a braided suture subcutaneously under and over the band, thereby looping the scar band. The sawing motion then releases the band without cutting the epidermis. Joseph Haik[32] introduced the technique, first used for releasing platysma bands, and extrapolated it to neck burn contracture release. The author expanded the use to all other body areas and conducted a retrospective study on 97 such releases (currently under review for publication). The overall satisfaction with the procedure was very good and the measurable increase in range of motion was significant (measured by independent occupational therapists). The contracture bands do not re-form, rather, the patients notice other, previously not noticed, "bands" that can be released subsequently. It can be safely applied in any body area that demonstrates appropriate subcutaneous scar bands to relieve the feeling of tightness and ideally increase of range of motion. Underlying major vascular or nerve structures need to be mapped and avoided prior to this intervention.

Lymphedema is an unresolved problem for burn survivors. Be it through constricting scars or fascial excision. There often is a profound derangement of the lymphatic system. Compression therapy has been the mainstay of therapy. With newer treatment options for lymphedema in other conditions like cancer treatment–related disturbance of lymphatic flow, there is hope that these techniques can be applied to burn reconstruction.[33] These include lymph node transplantation and new pathway creation by microvascular techniques.[33]

SUMMARY

Combined with advanced dermal substrates, spray-on skin and the development of fractional lasers are probably the most critical recent technologies in burn care and reconstruction. Regenerative medicine advances are leading to self-assembling whole skin substrates, which will revolutionize the treatment of skin injuries shortly. Emerging technologies in other fields of medicine spill over into burn treatment and reconstruction. Interdisciplinary cooperation is essential in driving the developments forward and making them available to burn patients. Close cooperation with development institutions and engineering entities is instrumental.

In desperate need are long-term outcome studies of all these described interventions. Only large national and possibly international data collections like the breast cancer and reconstruction database will eventually be able to determine the value of individual burn care and reconstruction treatments.[34]

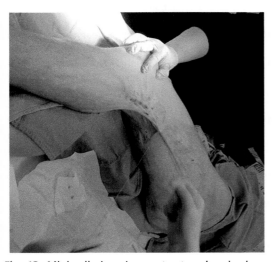

Fig. 13. Minimally invasive contracture band release on a knee contracture.

CLINICS CARE POINTS

- Consider burn eschar removal on hands, feet, face, and neck by enzymatic debridement.
- Consider coverage with dermal regeneration substrate of burns that reach past dermal elements.
- Employ advanced epidermal skin substitutes for pain control and scar prevention.
- Employ autologous cell spray to decrease donor sites and improve outcomes.
- Employ state-of-the-art diagnostic tools to determine burn depth and perfusion of tissue.
- Abstain from traditional skin grafting of burns with remaining dermal element and scar excision. Instead, use autologous cell spray and scar remodeling techniques like lasers and microneedling to modify and remodel the existing scar, often while preserving sensation and contour and pigmentation.

DISCLOSURE

The author has nothing to disclose.

REFERENCES

1. Janzekovic Z. A new concept in the early excision and immediate grafting of burns. J Trauma 1970; 10(12):1103–8.
2. Miotke SA. 107 the pioneering work of Dr. Zora Janzekovic. J Burn Care Res 2018;39(suppl_1):S59.
3. Liu H, Yue K, Cheng S, et al. A framework for automatic burn image segmentation and burn depth diagnosis using deep learning. Comput Math Methods Med 2021;2021:5514224.
4. Rowland R, Ponticorvo A, Baldado M, et al. Burn wound classification model using spatial frequency-domain imaging and machine learning. J Biomed Opt 2019;24(5):1–9.
5. Jaspers MEH, van Haasterecht L, van Zuijlen PPM, et al. A systematic review on the quality of measurement techniques for the assessment of burn wound depth or healing potential. Burns 2018;45(2):261–81.
6. Salinas J, Chung KK, Mann EA, et al. Computerized decision support system improves fluid resuscitation following severe burns: an original study. Crit Care Med 2011;39(9):2031–8.
7. Practice guidelines for moderate procedural sedation and analgesia 2018: a report by the American society of Anesthesiologists task force on moderate procedural sedation and analgesia, the American association of oral and maxillofacial surgeons, American college of radiology, American dental association, American society of dentist Anesthesiologists, and society of interventional radiology. Anesthesiology 2018;128(3):437–79.
8. Hirche C, Kreken Almeland S, Dheansa B, et al. Eschar removal by bromelain based enzymatic debridement (Nexobrid®) in burns: European consensus guidelines update. Burns 2020;46(4): 782–96.
9. Eriksson E, Grossman P, Pittinger T, et al. Consensus on the benefits of the exsurco medical amalgatome SD in the treatment of burns and other wounds. Eplasty 2019;19:b5.
10. Rheinwald JG, Green H. Serial cultivation of strains of human epidermal keratinocytes: the formation of keratinizing colonies from single cells. Cell 1975; 6(3):331–43.
11. Kowal S, Kruger E, Bilir P, et al. Cost-effectiveness of the use of autologous cell harvesting device compared to standard of care for treatment of severe burns in the United States. Adv Ther 2019; 36(7):1715–29.
12. Moiemen N, Schiestl C, Hartmann-Fritsch F, et al. First time compassionate use of laboratory engineered autologous Zurich skin in a massively burned child. Burns Open 2021;5(3):113–7.
13. Quintero EC, Machado JFE, Robles RAD. Meek micrografting history, indications, technique, physiology and experience: a review article. J Wound Care 2018;27(Sup2):S12–8.
14. Chogan F, Chen Y, Wood F, et al. Skin tissue engineering advances in burns: a brief introduction to the past, the present, and the future potential. J Burn Care Res 2023;44(Suppl_1):S1–4.
15. Halim AS, Khoo TL, Mohd Yussof SJ. Biologic and synthetic skin substitutes: an overview. Indian J Plast Surg 2010;43(Suppl):S23–8.
16. Hayashida K, Akita S. Surgical treatment algorithms for post-burn contractures. Burns Trauma 2017;5:9.
17. Blome-Eberwein S, Gogal C, Weiss MJ, et al. Prospective evaluation of fractional CO2 laser treatment of mature burn scars. J Burn Care Res 2016;37(6): 379–87.
18. Nuri T, Ueda K, Fujimori Y. Ten-year follow-up after treating extended burn scar contracture with an autologous cultured dermal substitute. Plast Reconstr Surg Glob Open 2018;6(6):e1782.
19. Orgill DP, Ogawa R. Current methods of burn reconstruction. Plast Reconstr Surg 2013;131(5):827e–36e.
20. Kohlert S, Quimby AE, Saman M, et al. Postoperative free-flap monitoring techniques. Semin Plast Surg 2019;33(1):13–6.
21. Fredman R, Katz AJ, Hultman CS. Fat grafting for burn, traumatic, and surgical scars. Clin Plast Surg 2017;44(4):781–91.

22. Sohrabi C, Goutos I. The use of botulinum toxin in keloid scar management: a literature review. Scars Burn Heal 2020;6. 2059513120926628.

23. Hu L, Zou Y, Chang SJ, et al. Effects of botulinum toxin on improving facial surgical scars: a prospective, split-scar, double-blind, randomized controlled trial. Plast Reconstr Surg 2018;141(3):646–50.

24. Garner J, Davidson D, Eckert GJ, et al. Reshapable polymeric hydrogel for controlled soft-tissue expansion: in vitro and in vivo evaluation. J Control Release 2017;262:201–11.

25. Chummun S, Addison P, Stewart KJ. The osmotic tissue expander: a 5-year experience. J Plast Reconstr Aesthet Surg 2010;63(12):2128–32.

26. Sosin M, Ceradini DJ, Levine JP, et al. Total face, eyelids, ears, scalp, and skeletal subunit transplant: a reconstructive solution for the full face and total scalp burn. Plast Reconstr Surg 2016;138(1):205–19.

27. Dorante MI, Wang AT, Kollar B, et al. Facial expression after face transplant: an international face transplant cohort comparison. Plast Reconstr Surg 2023;152:315e–25e.

28. La Padula S, Pensato R, Pizza C, et al. Face transplant: indications, outcomes, and ethical issues-where do we stand? J Clin Med 2022;11(19):5750.

29. Diep GK, Berman ZP, Alfonso AR, et al. The 2020 facial transplantation update: a 15-year compendium. Plast Reconstr Surg Glob Open 2021;9(5):e3586.

30. Alster TS. Cutaneous resurfacing with CO_2 and erbium: YAG lasers: preoperative, intraoperative, and postoperative considerations. Plast Reconstr Surg 1999;103(2):619–32. discussion 633-4.

31. Klifto KM, Asif M, Hultman CS. Laser management of hypertrophic burn scars: a comprehensive review. Burns Trauma 2020;8:tkz002.

32. Haik J, Prat D, Kornhaber R, et al. Treatment of cervical contractures utilising a closed platysmotomy like approach: case report and review of the literature. Burns 2016;42(6):e93–7.

33. Park KE, Allam O, Chandler L, et al. Surgical management of lymphedema: a review of current literature. Gland Surg 2020;9(2):503–11.

34. Young A, Davies A, Tsang C, et al. Establishment of a core outcome set for burn care research: development and international consensus. BMJ Med 2022;1(1):e000183.

Acute and Reconstructive Burn Care of the Hand

Shanmuganathan Raja Sabapathy, MS, MCh, DNB, FRCS(Ed), FAMS, Hon FRCS (Glas), Hon FRCS (Eng) Hon FACS, D Sc (Hon)[a],[*],[1], R. Raja Shanmugakrishnan, MBBS, MS, MRCS, DNB[a],[b],[1], Charles Scott Hultman, MD, MBA[c]

KEYWORDS

• Acute burns • Postburn • Hand • Contracture • Reconstruction • Pedicled flap

KEY POINTS

- Functional integration of a burn patient into the society depends upon the functionality of the hands.
- Accurate assessment of the depth of the burns and appropriate treatment will prevent post-burn deformities.
- Outcome of deformity correction depends on extent of deformity correction obtained by surgery and maintained till wound healing.
- All deformity correction patients need long-term supervised physiotherapy.

INTRODUCTION

The hand is commonly affected in thermal injuries. Hand burns account for 39% of all burns and they are involved in 34% of instances when the total body surface area (TBSA) of a burn exceeds 15%.[1],[2] Inadequate or inappropriate treatment could result in significant morbidity. The ultimate integration of a burn patient into the society largely depends on the functionality of the hands. Hence, it is important to reduce complications by providing good care during the acute stage. If deformities occur, reconstructive surgery followed up with good physiotherapy can help restore function but could be demanding both on the surgeon and patient.

Anatomical Considerations

Function of the hand depends upon stability of the skeleton, gliding motion of the tendons, and intact sensate skin cover. Though burns often affect only the skin, the response to the injury and the anatomic derangements that take place in the acute and healing phase has the potential to cause severe disability. On the hand, the dorsal skin is much thinner than the palmar skin. For the hand to function fully, the dorsal skin must be non-adherent and elastic, allowing hand closure and the palmar skin must be thick enough to withstand forces arising from daily use. Dorsal hand burns are most often flame or explosion injuries; palmar burns occur more frequently from chemicals, friction, or high-voltage contacts.

The thick palmar skin is tightly held to the skeleton by fibrous septa while the dorsal skin is thin and loosely attached to the underlying structures.

Edema occurring in the acute post-burn period preferentially accumulates on the dorsum causing wrist flexion, extension of the metacarpophalangeal joints, and flexion of the interphalangeal joints (IP) joints causing a claw deformity (**Fig. 1**). That is also the position of comfort. We need to remember a burn treatment adage: The position of comfort is the position of deformity.[3] If left uncorrected, the contracted collateral ligaments of the metacarpophalangeal (MCP) joints and the shortened volar plate of the IP joints pose a challenge in correction.

[a] Department of Plastic Surgery, Hand & Reconstructive Microsurgery & Burns, Ganga Hospital, 313, Mettupalayam Road, Coimbatore, Tamil Nadu 641 043, India; [b] Department of Hand, Reconstructive Microsurgery, Faciomaxillary and Burns, Ganga Hospital, Coimbatore, Tamil Nadu, India; [c] WPP Plastic and Reconstructive Surgery, WakeMed Health and Hospitals, 3000 New Bern Avenue, Raleigh, NC 27610, USA
[1] Present address: Ganga Hospital, 313, Mettupalayam Road, Coimbatore, India - 641043
[*] Corresponding author. Ganga Hospital, 313, Mettupalayam Road, Coimbatore, India - 641043.
E-mail address: rajahand@gmail.com

Clin Plastic Surg 51 (2024) 365–377
https://doi.org/10.1016/j.cps.2024.02.007

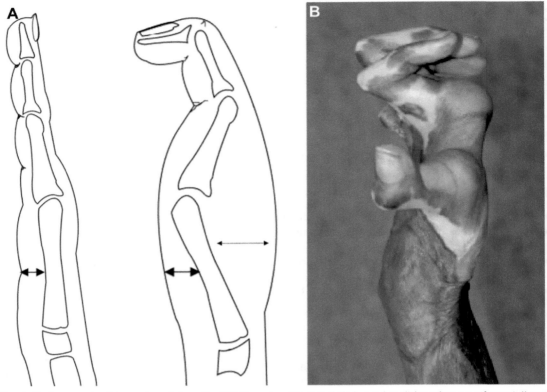

Fig. 1. Pathogenesis of burn claw deformity. (*A*) The volar skin is tightly bound and the edema preferentially collects on the dorsum causing hyperextension deformity at the metacarpophalangeal (MCP) joint. The adjacent joints take up the opposite position, (*B*) a fully formed deformity with flexion at the wrist, hyperextension at the MCP joints, and flexion at the proximal interphalangeal joint (PIP) joint.

A combination of deep dermal or deep burns and edema causes thinning or ulceration of the skin over the dorsum of the IP joints. Over the proximal interphalangeal (PIP) joints, it can cause attenuation or rupture of the central slip causing boutonniere deformity.

Edema fluid occurring on the palmar side is masked by the tight fibrous septa but nevertheless can cause significant problems. In deep circumferential burns of the hands or fingers, the unyielding leathery skin causes arterial insufficiency. It could also cause nerve compression in the carpal tunnel and Guyon canal and compartment syndrome. A combination of contracted intrinsics and contraction of the burn scars on the dorsum of the finger can result in swan neck deformity. The focus in acute care is to reduce edema in the acute phase and achieve healing as early as possible without resorting to secondary healing.

First Aid and Assessment of a Hand Burn

The aim is to douse the fire and reduce the effects of the thermal injury. Both are achieved by keeping the hand in flowing water until the patient feels comfortable. Tap water at room temperature is acceptable. This needs to be done for at least 20 minutes. Water rapidly reduces the subdermal temperature and prevents the burn injury from becoming deeper. Constricting items like rings and jewellery are to be removed immediately. If it is part of a major injury, all patients must be examined as per the Advanced Trauma Life Support (ATLS) protocol in order not to miss any associated injuries. Though the hand accounts for only 2% of TBSA, according to the American Burn Association, a burn of any depth to the hand is classified as a major injury and requires treatment at a specialized burn center.[4]

Extent and the depth of burns are the 2 important things that have to be decided upon during initial assessment. Depth assessment is important because other than superficial burns which could be left to heal spontaneously, hand burns deep dermal and deep burns have to be operated early to prevent inevitable contracture.

Redness, skin blanching under pressure, and area painful to air and temperature indicate superficial burn. Blisters when unroofed, revealing skin which is wet or waxy, dry with variable contour and skin which does not blanch on pressure denote deep dermal burn and in addition, if the area is waxy white or leathery gray, charred, dry, and inelastic with no blanching to pressure and if thrombosed veins are visible, then it is a deep burn.

At first assessment, the areas are marked on a diagram and photographs done before applying any ointment which may later make the assessment of depth difficult. In addition, the circulation of fingertips as assessed by blanching on pressure, sensation at the fingertip, and pain on passive extension of the fingers are noted for signs of compartment syndrome. These are important in case of electrical burns and circumferential burn injuries.

Acute Care in Special Type of Burns

Chemical Burns: The crucial difference between a chemical burn and a thermal burn is that the damage continues until the chemical is removed or neutralized.[5] Loose dry agents must be dusted off and clothing must be removed. Immediate high-volume water lavage is the treatment of choice, and it should last for at least 20 minutes and in cases of concentrated alkali can last for several hours. Use of neutralizing compounds or alternative lavage substances is generally discouraged. There are certain exceptions to the use of water. Phenol is insoluable in water, so polyethylene glycol may be used initially to increase its solubility in water. Elemental metals like sodium, potassium, and lithium combust when exposed to water; hence, burns from these metals should be immersed in mineral oil and the metal with the mineral oil is then removed. Dry lime becomes caustic only on contact with water and so it is dusted off.

The damage could be more severe than simple thermal burns. Good history and knowledge of the chemical involved and the concentration and duration of contact will be crucial. It is advisable to consult a specialist center and follow the protocols of management.

Electrical burns: Electrical injuries have been classified as high-voltage and low-voltage injuries (more and <1000 V respectively). Low-voltage injuries occur in the domestic environment while high-voltage injuries occur in the workplace. Both may be lethal.

In survivors, low-voltage injuries would need debridement and reconstruction of the local area, whereas high-voltage injuries need massive resuscitation efforts and intensive care in the acute phase.[6] Cardiac assessment for myocardial involvement, occurence of arrythmia and maintaining high-volume urine output are important.

Electrical burns cause severe edema and most will require fasciotomies and carpal tunnel decompression on arrival. Though there are techniques to measure compartment pressures, decision to decompress is clinical. Blood creatinine phosphokinase levels give an idea of the extent of muscle damage, but are also not a determinant of the need for fasciotomy.[7] If there is severe swelling of the forearm, and it feels tense, the patient will benefit from fasciotomy. The illustration of lines of incision are marked in the diagram (**Fig. 2**).[8] Later, they would need serial wound debridement and major reconstructive procedures.

Dressings for Hand Burns

After a decision is made on the depth of burns, if there are no indications for immediate surgery, dressings are done. The burnt area is dressed with topical agents. There are many topical agents available ranging from simple occlusive moist dressing to some with antibacterial properties. The authors prefer non adherent paraffin-soaked gauze. There are dressings with antibacterial properties and there is not much to choose from one another except the ease and frequency of application and cost. It is beyond the scope of this article to discuss all the available materials and the reader is referred to many articles which deal with this in detail[9,10]

The main aim of the dressing is to position the hand to reduce the edema, keep the fingertips visible for inspection, and facilitate movement. This is achieved by putting a conforming and comfortable dressing and putting a plaster slab on the initial day keeping the wrist in about 20° of extension, the

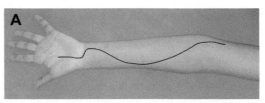

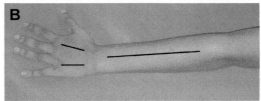

Fig. 2. Line of fasciotomy incisions: (*A*) Volar side. Staring with carpal tunnel decompression, the incision is extended proximally. The design is to prevent exposure of the median nerve. (*B*) Incisions on the dorsum to decompress extensors and the interossei in the hand. The mobile wad is to be decompressed through either of the incisions.

MCP joints in about 60 to 80° of flexion, and the IP joints in as much of extension as possible. Though a 90-degree position of the MCP joint and neutral position of the IP joints is preferable, seldom is it possible to achieve it on day 1. In addition, the authors position the forearm in supination since it will help in rehabilitation. A forearm stiff in pronation, with the wrist stiff in flexion is severely nonfunctional and difficult to correct. The patient is encouraged to move the fingers. Elevation and movement are the two factors which reduce edema.

After a few days, special orthotic splints are made, with the wrist in 20° of dorsiflexion, MCP joints in 90° flexion, and the IP joints in extension. This is used whenever the patient is not moving the fingers and retained till healing of the wound. Dressing changes are made as per the topical agent used and before the application, the hand is washed with soap and water. Simple washing with soap and water reduces the bacterial colony count significantly.

Immediate Surgery in Hand Burns

In circumferential full thickness burns and deep partial thickness burns, edema can cause circulatory compromise. Ultrasound recordings, pulse oximetry, photoelectric plethysmography have been tried but escharotomy has to be done on clinical grounds. If the fingers or hand starts feeling cold and palmar arch pulse disappears on Doppler, it is better to decompress. Significant increase in survival of the fingers has been found following lateral digital escharotomy compared with those not decompressed.[11] Escharotomy is done on the ulnar side of the index, middle, ring, and little finger along the mid lateral line and carried proximally to hypothenar eminence. On the thumb, it is done on the radial side first.

If there is compartment syndrome, the fingers could take the posture of swan neck deformity with difficulty in flexing the PIP joint. The Finochietto test—difficulty to flex the proximal interphalangeal joint (PIP) joint with the MCP joint placed in hyperextension—will be positive. The thenar, hypothenar, and interossei muscles have to be decompressed. If the sensation is reduced and clawing is present, it is a sign of nerve compression and warrants carpal tunnel and Guyon canal decompression. This is common in electrical burns of the hand and the authors have found that even after decompression, it might take a few weeks for clawing to disappear (Fig. 3).

Early Surgery for Hand Burns

Early surgery in hand burns is done in deep dermal, full thickness, and fourth-degree burns.

Tangential Excision for deep dermal burns: Early tangential excision and immediate cover of burns was initiated by Zora Janžekovič.[12] It involves shaving of the burnt superficial part of the skin leaving back the unburnt dermis behind and covering it with thin split skin graft. It was based on her observation that many deep dermal burns did not end up with good outcomes on conservative management. In such cases, she found that the burnt superficial dermis got infected, and infection destroyed the uninvolved dermis converting the deep dermal to a full thickness burns. This is prevented by early tangential excision. In this process, the deep dermal burn is sequentially shaved in thin layers up to the level of viable dermis and covered with thin skin graft and they are known to give excellent functional outcomes (Fig. 4). Since some dermis is left behind, and the sweat glands and hair follicles are present, thin graft provides better results. Retention cysts which develop can just be brushed away. Thick grafts and widely meshed grafts give poor results after tangential excision of burns.

Burn wound excision: In full thickness burns, the burn wound is excised and depending upon the bed, skin graft or flap cover is provided. The excision could be only the skin or in deeper burns, sometimes it is done to the level of the fascia. While graft take is better with excision to fascia, it leaves behind an contour defect. While thin grafts are applied after tangential excision of deep dermal burns, after full thickness excision, moderately thick split thickness graft is applied. Thicker the graft the less are the chances of contraction.

Early reconstruction: Localized electrical burns are mostly deep burns and they require early excision and flap cover. Local or regional flaps can be used if the area is limited (Fig. 5). Though it can be done immediately, the authors usually do it by around the fifth day, when the local edema has settled and the extent of damage is also well delineated. The authors do not hesitate to use distant pedicled flaps or free flaps when the defects are large, or involve multiple fingers.

Physiotherapy Following Early Surgery

Edema control, early movement, massage with moisturising creams, and compression of the scar and grafted areas are the key elements of physiotherapy protocol following acute burn management.

Burns which heal within 14 days are superficial and the skin is almost restored to normal function. Contractures do not develop, and scarring is minimal. These patients need to apply moisturizing cream and do all normal work.

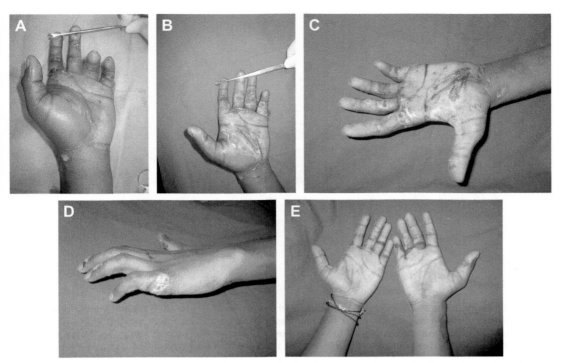

Fig. 3. (A) Electrical burns at presentation. The patient had reduced sensation at the fingertips and tendency to clawing is seen, (B) carpal and Guyon canal decompression done, (C, D) the hand at 3 weeks showing a full-blown total claw hand, (E) fully recovered at 3 months.

Patients whose burns have taken longer to heal or have undergone surgery or grafting will need scar management. The goal of scar management is to modulate scars as much as possible to achieve a flat, smooth, supple, and aesthetically acceptable scar, with no functional limitations. This is achieved by the effective use of compression dressings, silicone products, and massage[13–15]

Management of Post Burn Contractures

Though it is ideal to prevent the post burn contractures, inadequate primary care either due to logistic reasons or when hand burns form part of a major burn predisposes to deformities. It can affect any joint and could seriously limit function. Many classifications exist to describe the extent of the contractures in individual joints.[16–19] In the authors' experience, the authors have found that barring minor contractures, burn deformities affect multiple joints to different extents and it becomes difficult to classify them. Though it is good to classify, a good descriptive and photographic documentation has been found to be more useful. With that the authors use scores like Disabilities of the Arm, Shoulder and Hand (DASH) and Mental Health Quotient (MHQ) to assess pre-functional and post-functional status.

At Ganga Hospital, the authors apply the following principles when they manage post burn contractures of the hand[20]

1. While reconstructing a burnt hand, the burn surgeon must concentrate on restoring function

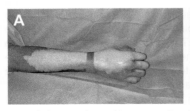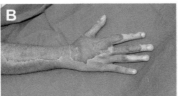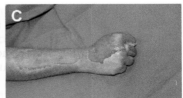

Fig. 4. (A) Deep dermal burns on the dorsum of hand, fingers, and forearm, (B, C) Outcome of tangential excision done with application of thin skin graft.

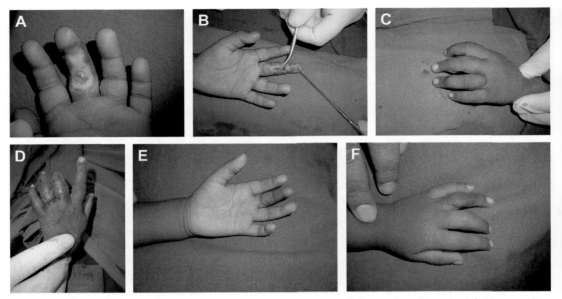

Fig. 5. (A) Low-voltage electrical burns of the finger with exposure of the tendon, (B) early debridement done, showing the extent of skin loss, (C) a large cross-finger flap marked on the dorsum of the ring finger, (D) flap inset and the donor area covered with skin graft, (E, F) long-term outcome. The patient had good flexion and extension. Over time, the flap develops crease at the level of the PIP joint due to good flexion.

than on increasing the range of movement of individual joints.

Surgery on the burnt hand must restore pinch, the ability to grasp large objects, and the power grip. This is obtained when the thumb pulp meets the pulp of other fingers, the hand has adequate first web space, and the musculotendinous units function to provide adequate power. Surgical procedures must be chosen to achieve these, rather than aiming for an increase in the range of movement in each individual joint. For example, it might be an advantage to have a PIP joint arthrodesed in good functional position than to perform complicated procedures to restore movement in a bad boutonniere deformity.

2. When a hand is severely involved, choose the first set of procedures that will bring the maximum benefit to the patient.

It is usual for a severe burn contracture to undergo a series of procedures to obtain the ultimate functional result, but the first procedure must produce a perceivable improvement in function. Early restoration of independence in the use of the hand will boost the morale and encourage the patient to adhere to postoperative protocols and take up subsequent procedures.

When contractures occur at multiple joints, correction usually starts from proximal to distal unless the proximal deformities are minor.

3. Assess the deformity in each tissue component to make the treatment plan.

Burn deformities occur secondary to skin loss. But deformity correction involves not only correcting the skin loss but also the secondary changes that have occurred in the musculotendinous units and joints. They usually are the limiting factors for deformity correction. Evaluate the deformity in each of the components of skin, tendons, joints, and bones while making the treatment plan.

4. Success in deformity correction depends on the excision of the scar tissue and correcting the deforming forces than on the type of skin cover provided.

Most deformity correction would need skin replacement. Mere replacement of the burn scar with skin graft or a flap will not correct the burn deformity. The deformity must first be corrected to achieve thumb-finger opposition, wide first web space, and flexion at the MCP joints and then the defect be planned for soft tissue cover. The correction achieved on the table is the maximum that could be achieved. Therapists have to work hard to maintain the gains of surgery and cannot be expected to provide more correction than what was achieved on the table.

5. Timing of surgery is crucial to get a good outcome in deformity correction. It is better to perform the surgery when there is tissue

equilibrium, as shown by a reduction of the induration and the scars becoming pale.

While this principle holds good for most instances, the authors prefer early correction of deformities in children. Scars in young children can deform bones and cause dislocation of joints. Articular cartilages retain their vitality only when they are in contact with another smooth articular surface and enclosed in a joint capsule and bathed by synovial fluid. When the joints remain dislocated for long, the surface loses its sheen and vitality and restitution of congruous joint surfaces still may not restore good function.

6. Function is very important, but a burn surgeon must also constantly think of the aesthetic aspect of reconstruction of a burned hand.

The hand is a part that is always exposed and constantly reminds the patient that he is different. An aesthetically acceptable reconstruction helps him or her to easily integrate back into the society. The statement that "hand surgery is also aesthetic surgery" has never been truer than in the treatment of burned hands.

7. Physiotherapy, splinting, and scar control measures are important to achieve good outcome. Supervised physiotherapy at least for 8 weeks after reconstruction is essential after any major reconstruction.

All these principles will apply to the correction of any burn deformity in some way or the other.

Technical Note on Specific Deformities

Burn Syndactyly: Burns to the dorsum of the fingers usually also affect the sides of the fingers. If allowed to heal secondarily or if the grafts do not take fully, syndactyly results. It affects lateral pinch when the index is involved and reduces the span of holding an object. Conventionally, it is advised that during correction, we need to plan a flap of normal skin in the web. In burns, most often it will not be possible. Good outcome is achieved by painstakingly suturing the grafts ensuring full take of the graft. Post healing, the authors use silicone sheets taped to the web (Fig. 6) and maintained for about 6 months. Silicone must not be applied to raw areas or unstable scar. Moderate thick split skin graft is to be used.

First web contracture: The first web is a specialized anatomic entity, triangular in outline with the apex between the bases of the first and second metacarpals and a thin base distally. Only band contracture of the skin at the free edge is amenable to correction by various forms of Z-plasty.[21] In most instances, there is always a shortage of skin and

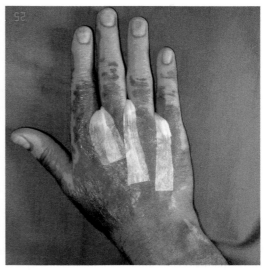

Fig. 6. Technique of compression of the graft after web reconstruction with skin graft. A small strip of silicone sheet is placed and secured with plaster tapes.

there must be no hesitation in adding up skin to replace the lost skin.

With long-standing severe contractures, the first dorsal interossei and the adductor pollicis undergo adaptive shortening. To release the web, the first dorsal interossei must be released from its origin from the first metacarpal and the adductor pollicis must be released from the third metacarpal. In this way, they retain their innervation, form a new attachment, and continue to have adequate function.

Circumduction movement at the carpometacarpal (CMC) joint of the thumb is important for pulp pinch and opposition.[22] This is achieved by releasing the tight skin on the dorsum of the CMC joint by a transverse incision. The transverse incision could be continued volar across the wrist.

The released thumb is stabilized in full abduction in line with the outer border of the index finger by a K-wire passing as a spacer between the first and second metacarpal. The wire is retained for about 3 weeks till the wound healing is complete and the patient is ready to start physiotherapy. The tendency to stabilize the thumb in extension must be resisted. Thumb in an extended position would lead to inadequate skin replacement. If release needs more than skin release, flap would be needed. In isolated hand burns, posterior interosseous flap is a good choice. Otherwise, the authors usually prefer a groin flap or a free lateral arm flap (Fig. 7).

Dorsal contracture release

Dorsal hand contractures are sometimes associated with volar contractures of the wrist and IP

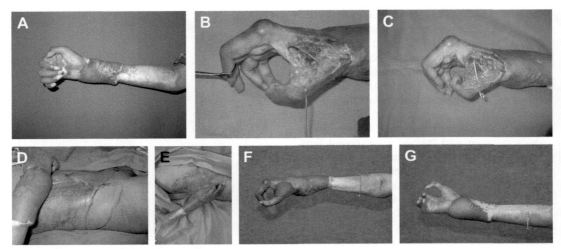

Fig. 7. (A) Severe contracture of the first web space in an electrical burn, (B) picture at the completion of web release, (C) the release obtained is maintained by a transverse K-wire passed between the first and second metacarpals. (D) Marking of the groin flap, (E) inset of the flap, (F, G) long-term pictures showing preservation of the web space.

joints and first web contractures. If present, they have to be released first or along with dorsal contracture release. The goal of dorsal contracture release is to obtain flexion at the MCP joints. A transverse incision is made a few centimeters proximal to the MCP joint line. This is to make allowance for migration of the skin after release so that it will cover the MCP joint after capsulotomy. The scar is excised, tenolysis of the extensors are done and if necessary, tendons lengthened.

The MCP joint can be approached for capsulotomy underneath the flap. The extensor expansion is split in the midline and the joint released. But the authors found that in long-standing contractures on attempting flexion post-surgery, it causes opening up of the sutures. Hence, the authors prefer to approach the joint by going beneath the sagittal bands and with the use of the curved tenotomy scissors divide the capsule and the contracted collateral ligaments. Post release, the joint is pinned till wound healing.

In long-standing extension contractures, the MCP joints may be subluxated or dislocated. During reduction, a volar pocket has to be made for the articular surface of the proximal phalanx to slide over the head of the metacarpal.[23] If it is not achieved, the joint surfaces go back and recurrence of contracture is inevitable (**Fig. 8**).

A component of the dorsal extension contracture of the MCP joints is flattening of the transverse arch of the palm. Longitudinal skin release incisions are made in the web which will spread out to regain the cupping of the palm.

Post release, the choice of skin cover is made on the basis of the nature of the defect. If the defect would accept a graft, the authors prefer a medium thickness graft. Small areas of exposure of the tendons can be managed with the application of dermal substitutes and later skin grafting. If bare tendons or joints are exposed, the authors opt for a flap. Pedicled groin or lower abdominal flaps or free flaps can be used to cover the defect (**Fig. 9**).

Palmar Contracture: Contracture of the palm occurs less often than dorsum and is more common in chemical, electrical, and in certain religious practices. The skin of the palm is thicker and most often heals without skin graft. But if there is skin loss, it has to be taken care of since contractures are more difficult to correct. Dorsal contractures even if they are long standing, do not have the risk of shortened vessels and nerves. On the other hand, contracture of the palm and flexion contracture of the fingers have the serious risk of stretching of the nerves and vessels compromising their integrity during release.

While releasing palm contracture, attention is also drawn to the adduction contracture of the thumb. Skin grafts are the preferred option so that the cupping of the palm is maintained, and good grip is possible (**Fig. 10**). If a flap cover must be given, a thin flap has to be chosen. A bulky flap makes prehension difficult and has to be thinned early.

Finger Contractures: Flexion contractures of the fingers are common and frequently accompany extension contracture of the MCP joints (**Fig. 11**).

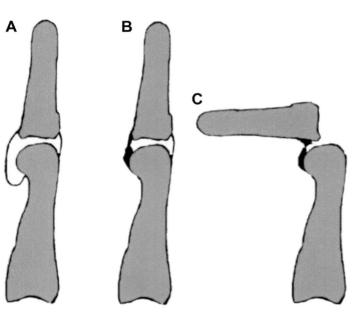

Fig. 8. (*A*) Normal MCP joint, which has a synovial laxity for the gliding of the base of the proximal phalanx over the head of the metacarpal. (*B*) In extension burn contracture, the volar capsule is contracted and scarred preventing gliding of the proximal phalanx over the head of the metacarpal. (*C*) If the pouch is not recreated during release, the proximal phalanx buckles up and it will cause sure recurrence of the deformity.

Finger flexion contractures need to be released first since early extension contracture release of the MCP joints will make the fingertips bury into the palm. Minor band contractures are released by Z- plasty. In fingers, it is good to keep the flaps of the Z big and the tip a bit broad so that good release is obtained, the flaps are viable, and suturing is easy.

Correction of severe contractures would need skin replacement. Contractures are released by cutting across the contractures. Critical structures like vessels, tendons, and nerves have a tendency to get exposed at the level of the joint. In contractures of moderate severity, release is done by incisions on either side of the joint line leaving a small bipedicle flap in between over the joint and grafting on either side. This yields better results than a flap. If the tendon gets exposed in a small area, the bipedicle flap can be used to cover as a transposition flap by dividing one end and the raw area grafted.

If the contractures are very severe, full release and full thickness graft or a flap is needed. Single fingers can be managed by cross finger flaps and other local flaps. If multiple fingers are

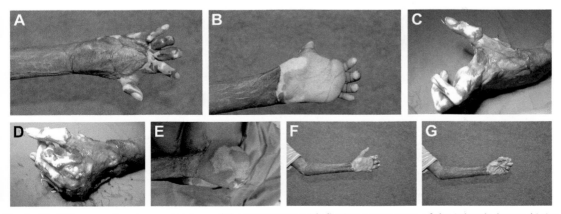

Fig. 9. (*A, B*) Severe extension contracture of the MCP joints with flexion contracture of the interphalangeal joint (IP) joints and swan neck deformity of the thumb with total loss of function. (*C*) The extent of release of the thumb and positioning for flap cover, (*D*) position after release of the MCP joints. Note that the boutonniere deformity in the index and middle is not corrected, (*E*) the raw area is covered with a combined groin and hypogastric pedicled flap, (*F, G*) showing the thumb meeting the fingers and appreciable function in a single step.

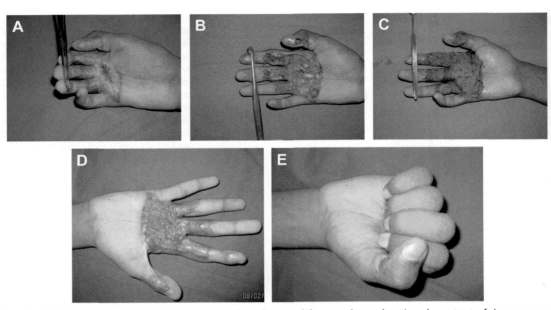

Fig. 10. (A) Contracture of the palm and base of the fingers, (B) post release showing the extent of the raw area, (C) coverage of the raw area with moderate thickness split skin graft, (D, E) long-term result showing excellent function.

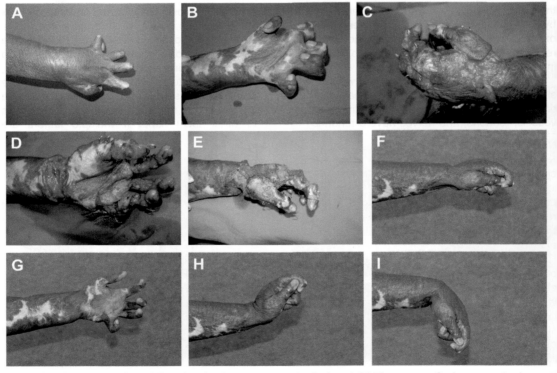

Fig. 11. (A, B) Severe combined dorsal and volar contracture in the hand. (C) The extent of release required to get the thumb to functional position. The arrow shows the area that has to be released to get protonation and op-position movement (circumduction) at the carpometacarpal joint of the thumb. (D) These patients almost always need release on the volar aspect of the wrist, which is the continuation of the incision at the base of the thumb. (E) All raw areas are covered with split skin graft, (F–I) pictures' of the functional outcome after 1 procedure.

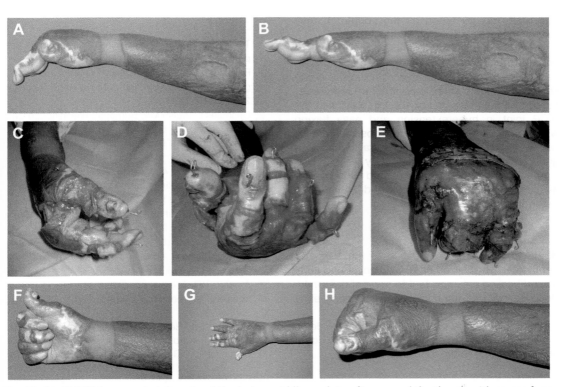

Fig. 12. (*A, B*) Stiff Swan neck deformity of the index, middle, and ring fingers and the thumb with severe functional compromise. (*C, D*) Multiple dorsal skin release done and (*E*) raw area covered with split skin graft. (*F–H*) Long-term functional result.

involved, temporary surgical syndactyly is made, and a flap cover is given.

Vascular compromise is a real risk while releasing flexion contractures of the fingers. Caution is to be exercised while stretching the joints during release. Normally, the released IP joints are stabilized with K-wires. Tourniquet is let down and vascularity confirmed before taking on the next step. If there is any doubt, as shown by the finger remaining pale or taking a long time to perfuse, the wire is removed, the joint gently flexed to the point where the circulation picks up, and the joint is stabilized at that level.

Boutonniere Deformity: Boutonniere deformity occurs due to dorsal burns causing severe edema at the level of the PIP joint. Poor positioning of the wrist and the MCP joints may result in flexed position of the IP joints for a long time. This causes stretching of the joint capsule and the attachment of the central slip leading to its attenuation and rupture. Further direct involvement of the overlying skin again could be a cause.

Pinning of the PIP joint in neutral position during the acute stage can be done to prevent boutonniere deformity. Position is maintained till wound healing occurs.

Once the deformity occurs, if the deformity is passively correctable, the PIP joint is splinted in extension and flexion at the distal interphalangeal (DIP) joint is encouraged. Later, if there is good dorsal skin, the joint is explored and correction surgeries are done.[24] This is only rarely possible in burns since the dorsal skin is scarred and thinned out and the patients present in a state of stiff joints.

Burn patients with stiff boutonniere deformity surprisingly retain good function since pinch is possible, if there is good MCP joint function. So the decision to correct is taken after assessing overall function. It may be prudent to arthrodese the PIP joint in functional position than suggesting complex deformity correction procedures.

Swan neck deformity: Unlike boutonniere deformity, swan neck deformity compromises function and correction is usually recommended. The commonest cause is contraction and hypertrophy of the dorsal skin over the fingers causing hyperextension deformity at the PIP joint and flexion at the DIP joint. Correction is done by incising the scarred skin on the dorsum on either side of the PIP joints, mobilizing the joints, stabilizing the PIP joint in flexed functional position, and grafting the raw areas.

The grafts contract and as they contract, they stretch the intervening skin bridge (**Fig. 12**).

The other cause of swan neck deformity is secondary to contracture of the intrinsic muscles as part of the compartment syndrome in the acute stage. Finochito's intrinsic contracture test (resistance and tightness to flex the PIP joint with the MCP joint in hyperextension and easy flexion with the MCP joints in a flexed position) will be positive. Division of the tight lateral bands is a good option to correct the deformity.

A good clinical assessment and judgment is needed to manage swan neck and boutonniere deformities.

SUMMARY

Burns to the hand irrespective of the size and depth need specialized care. Skin cover and early wound healing are important to prevent deformity. Deep dermal and full thickness burns need early surgery.

When contractures occur, attention to detail while planning and executing the procedure could be life changing to the individual.

CLINICS CARE POINTS

- All hand burns need to be seen by a specialist unit.
- Accurate assessment of the depth of hand burns and appropriate management will prevent deformity.
- During correction of post burn deformity, concentrate on gaining function than on range of movement of individual joints
- The extent of correction obtained at the end of surgery will be the maximum correction obtained and so go for full extent.
- Deformity correction must be undertaken early in children since secondary deformities are severe in children.
- All patients need long-term physiotherapy for scar control and maintaining the gains of surgery

DISCLOSURE

There are no disclosures.

FUNDING

There were no funding/ grants received.

REFERENCES

1. Tredget EE. Management of the acutely burned upper extremity. Hand Clin 2000;16(2):187–203.
2. Richards WT, Vergara E, Dalaly DG, et al. Acute surgical management of hand burns. J Hand Surg Am 2014;39(10):2075–85.e2.
3. Deshaies L, Walsh MA. Burns. In: Wietlishcach CM, editor. Cooper's Fundamentals of hand Therapy. 3rd edition. St Louis (Mo): Elsevier; 2020. p. 404–15.
4. American Burn Association/American College of Surgeons. Guidelines for the operation of burn centers. J Burn Care Res 2007;28(1):134–41.
5. Robinson EP, Chhabra AB. Hand chemical burns. J Hand Surg Am 2015;40(3):605–13.
6. Daniel RK, Ballard PA, Heroux P, et al. High-voltage electrical injury: acute pathophysiology. J Hand Surg Am 1988;13(1):44–9.
7. Arnoldo BD, Purdue GF. The diagnosis and management of electrical injuries. Hand Clin 2009; 25(4):469–79.
8. Norbury WB, Herndon DN. Management of acute pediatric hand burns. Hand Clin 2017;33(2):237–42.
9. Greenhalgh DG. Topical antimicrobial agents for burn wounds. Clin Plast Surg 2009;36(4):597–606.
10. Pan BS, Vu AT, Yakuboff KP. Management of the acutely burned hand. J Hand Surg Am 2015;40(7): 1477–85.
11. Sykes PJ. Severe burns of the hand. A Practical Guide in their management. J Hand Surg 1991; 16B:6–12.
12. Janzekovic Z. A new concept in the early excision and immediate grafting of burns. J Trauma 1970; 10(12):1103–8.
13. Ault P, Plaza A, Paratz J. Scar massage for hypertrophic burns scarring-A systematic review. Burns 2018;44(1):24–38.
14. Nedelec B, Carter A, Forbes L, et al. Practice guidelines for the application of nonsilicone or silicone gels and gel sheets after burn injury. J Burn Care Res 2015;36(3):345–74.
15. Ai JW, Liu JT, Pei SD, et al. The effectiveness of pressure therapy (15-25 mmHg) for hypertrophic burn scars: a systematic review and meta-analysis. Sci Rep 2017;7:40185.
16. McCauley RL. Reconstruction of the pediatric burned hand. Hand Clin 2009;25(4):543–50.
17. Gulgonen A, Ozer K. The correction of postburn contractures of the second through fourth web spaces. J Hand Surg Am 2007;32(4):556–64.
18. Graham TJ, Stern PJ, True MS. Classification and treatment of postburn metacarpophalangeal joint extension contractures in children. J Hand Surg Am 1990;15(3):450–6.
19. Stern PJ, Neale HW, Graham TJ, et al. Classification and treatment of postburn proximal interphalangeal

joint flexion contractures in children. J Hand Surg Am 1987;12(3):450–7.

20. Sabapathy SR, Bajantri B, Bharathi RR. Management of post burn hand deformities. Indian J Plast Surg 2010;43(Suppl):S72–9.

21. Brown M, Chung KC. Postburn contractures of the hand. Hand Clin 2017;33(2):317–31.

22. Greyson MA, Wilkens SC, Sood RF, et al. Five essential principles for first web space reconstruction in the burned hand. Plast Reconstr Surg 2020;146(5): 578e–87e.

23. Sabapathy SR. Hand burns. In: Sarabahi S, Tiwari VK, Goel A, et al, editors. Principles and practice of burn care. New Delhi (India): Jaypee Brothers Medical Publishers; 2010. p. 362–82.

24. Groenevelt F, Schoorl R. Reconstructive surgery of the post-burn boutonnière deformity. J Hand Surg Br 1986;11(1):23–30.

Pediatric Burns
From Acute Care Through Reconstruction in 2024

Mark D. Fisher, MD[a,b,*], William Norbury, MD, MBBS[a]

KEYWORDS

• Pediatric • Burns • Reconstruction • Resuscitation • Contractures

KEY POINTS

- The developing child has distinctive characteristics including the body, intellect, and heart.
- Each of these must be understood as the burn team seeks to provide expert acute and reconstructive care.
- In the following text, the authors focus on acute pediatric burn epidemiology, resuscitation, management of inhalational injury, and metabolism.
- Major burns derail the child in their developmental journey.
- Good pediatric burn reconstruction seeks to set the child back on track in the most efficient, patient-centered fashion.

INTRODUCTION

Burn injury remains among the top 10 causes of unintentional injury and death in children.[1]

In the 1950s, a child with burns of 50% total body surface area (TBSA) would have an expected mortality of 50%;[2] today this same mortality can be seen in those with burns greater than 90% TBSA.[3] Despite the significant advancements made over the last 50 years, major burn injuries in children continue to require a high number of surgical procedures and hospital resources. The cause of injury differs between separate age groups with younger children and infants more likely to sustain scalds and older children to sustain significant flame injuries.[4,5] Scald burns are often related to an accident in the kitchen such as pulling on the handle of a pan on the stove top, or the cord of a kettle, and less likely are accidental or intentional immersion in hot baths.[6] Immersion into a hot bathtub is another cause of both accidental and non-accidental injury in children.

In addition to early fluid resuscitation, prompt excision and grafting, meticulous control of infections, modulation of the hypermetabolic response. and management of any inhalation injury, specific expertise in the management of the psychological impact of the injury is required in pediatric patients to give the best outcomes.[7,8]

Initial Evaluation

Firstly, remove the child from the source of injury, take off affected clothing and jewelry then flush the area with cool water for 20 minutes.[9] This can help to reduce propagation of the injury, reduce edema and inflammation, inhibit the release of oxygen free radicals, and improve local wound microcirculation.[10] For small burns, the principles of initial care include analgesia, cooling, and covering.[11]

[a] Department of Plastic and Reconstructive Surgery, The Johns Hopkins University School of Medicine, Johns Hopkins Burn Center, 4940 Eastern Avenue Suite, P3-4-11, JHBMC Pavilion Building, Baltimore, MD 21224, USA; [b] Bayview Adult Burn Center
* Corresponding author. Johns Hopkins Burn Center, 4940 Eastern Avenue, 3rd Floor Suite P3-4-11, Pavilion Building, Baltimore, MD 21224.
E-mail address: markfisher@jhmi.edu
Twitter: @markdfishermd (W.N.)

Clin Plastic Surg 51 (2024) 379–390
https://doi.org/10.1016/j.cps.2024.02.008

However, care should be taken to prevent hypothermia in large TBSA burns; in such cases, once the burning process is stopped, the patient should be kept warm with clean (sterile, if possible) sheets or blankets. In cases of chemical injury, the area should be flushed with water for a minimum of 30 mins—if the chemical is in powder form then it should be brushed off the patient prior to irrigation.

Burn patients, pediatric or adult, with >10% TBSA burned should be assumed to be trauma patients and managed as such using the principles of Advance Trauma Life Support, any potentially life-threatening injuries should be identified and treated.

- Assess airway and administer 100% oxygen, obtain arterial blood gases and carboxyhemoglobin levels.[12]
- Assess for stridor, tachypnea, and hoarseness as they could indicate impending airway difficulties requiring immediate intubation.
- Assessment of chest wall excursion: if circumferential full thickness burns to the chest wall are present and ventilation is compromised then escharotomy of the chest should be performed.
- Blood pressure monitoring: if all extremities are involved, then invasive monitoring is preferred. Radial arterial lines are less reliable in pediatric patients, where a femoral arterial line is recommended.
- Urinary catheter: allowing a measure of end-organ function and hence a guide to adjust resuscitation fluids.
- Nasogastric tube: to alleviate gastric ileus
- Intensive care unit admission: TBSA >10%; inhalational injury with obvious or potential airway involvement; altered mental status or shock; circumferential burns compromising respiration or limb perfusion; impending or established compartment syndrome of limbs or abdomen; evidence of evolving organ dysfunction; or associated major trauma.[13]

Regular re-evaluation during the resuscitation period is the key to success; a persistent tachycardia or low urine output should alert the clinician to the possibility of a missed injury or under-resuscitation.

Resuscitation

Delays in starting resuscitation of burned patients result in worse outcomes; this is especially important in children as fluid losses are proportionally larger due to their low body weight to body surface area ratio. Therefore, intravenous (IV) access needs to be obtained immediately for all burns involving more than 15% TBSA and resuscitation is commenced. Two large-bore peripheral IV lines are adequate for resuscitation; they may be placed through burned skin, but must be secured to prevent accidental removal. Central access may also be obtained if peripheral access is problematic; internal jugular, subclavian, or femoral can be used. If all attempts at vascular access fail, then the intraosseous route is also an option and can be used in children of any age;[14–16] preferred sites for access being the anterior tibial plateau, medial malleolus, anterior iliac crest, and distal femur. Once access has been gained, the needle should be secured to prevent inadvertent dislodgement. Fluids administered via an interosseous route are allowed to drip in under gravity alone.

Several formulas are available for the calculation of fluid resuscitation; however, these should be viewed as a starting point and the final amounts given should be titrated to an assessment of adequate resuscitation. The standard "rule of nines" can be of use in making calculations for larger adolescents but is less useful in young children as the relative size of different body parts is different.[17]

There remains no consensus on the threshold at which IV resuscitation should be commenced in children, with some centers initiating at 10% and others at 20% TBSA. The exact fluids given, amounts of fluid, and end points such as urine output all remain an area of research. When calculating the volume of fluid required in adult burn patients, the standard Parkland formula is widely used with great success. However, it is less useful in young children as it can underestimate requirements in children with smaller burns and overestimate fluids in children with larger burns.[18] Therefore, children with large surface area burns should be resuscitated based on formulas calculated according to body surface area (BSA). Either a standard nomogram or formula can be used to calculate the BSA. Then, a formula such as the Galveston formula can be used to estimate fluid requirements more accurately: 5000 mL/m^2 TBSA burned plus 2000 mL/m^2 TBSA for maintenance fluid given over the first 24 hours after burn, with half the volume administered during the initial 8 hours and the second half given over the following 16 hours.[19] Subsequent fluid requirements are estimated at 3750 mL/m^2 TBSA burned for remaining open wounds plus 1500 mL/m^2 TBSA for maintenance requirements, reducing over time as the patient achieves wound coverage. While these calculations are being made and during the initial assessment, the following can be used as a guide for patients with visibly large burns, based on age.

- ≤5 year old: 125 mL lactated Ringers (LR) per hour
- 6 to 13 year old: 250 mL LR per hour
- >14 years: 500 mL LR per hour.

Type of fluid: Intravenous resuscitation fluid should be isotonic and be supplemented to replace electrolyte disturbances. Lactated Ringer's solution is the most commonly used resuscitation solution for the first 24 hours after burn. Small children and especially those under the age of 1 should also receive a separate maintenance dextrose fluid solution to prevent hypoglycemia as their glycogen stores are limited.

Electrolyte disturbances.

- Hyponatremia: often seen in first 48 hours, frequent monitoring and supplementation due to higher urinary sodium losses.
- Hypokalemia: replaced with oral potassium phosphate
- Hypocalcemia and hypomagnesemia also need regular surveillance and supplementation.

Assessment of Resuscitation

Routine assessment of volume status includes pulse pressure, mental status, distal extremity color, and capillary refill. However, an indwelling urinary drainage catheter is essential to monitor resuscitation in burns ≥20% TBSA. During the early phase of resuscitation, urine output should be assessed hourly, and the resuscitation fluid adjusted accordingly. Goals for urine output should be titrated to achieve a urine output of 1 mL/kg/h in children and 2 mL/kg/h in infants. If needed, initial fluid boluses should be administered in amounts appropriate to the size of the child and should be less than 25% of the total blood volume (20 mL/kg). Measurement of arterial blood gas pH with a base deficit or increase in lactic acid is of particular importance in this age group, reflecting decreased tissue perfusion. Trending these levels can help to guide further resuscitation measures.

The likelihood of over-resuscitation can be reduced by using formulas based on body surface area. However, this is a common occurrence leading to pulmonary edema, right heart failure, cerebral edema, and compartment syndrome of the extremities and abdomen. Assessment of cardiac function with transthoracic echocardiogram should be used early in those children who are not responding to standard resuscitation measures. Low compliance of the child's heart reduces the ability to increase stroke volume, so output depends on heart rate alone. If over-loaded, then de-resuscitation should be considered with fluid restriction and diuretics.

Inhalation Injury and Airway Management

Initial assessment of the airway of a child is of paramount importance due to the much smaller diameter of the trachea, leading to an increased risk of airway obstruction. Signs of inhalation injury such as facial burns, soot in the nares or mouth, stridor, raspy breath sounds, altered mental status, or inability to speak in full sentences all indicate the possibility of an inhalation injury and potential need for intubation. Patients with an inhalation injury typically require more resuscitation fluids, and as such can gain delayed edema within the mucosa of the airway.

Indications for early intubation.

- Signs of airway obstruction: hoarseness, stridor, accessory respiratory muscle use, sternal retraction
- Extent of the burn (TBSA burn > 40%–50%)
- Extensive and deep facial burns
- Burns inside the mouth.
- Significant edema or risk for edema
- Difficulty swallowing
- Signs of respiratory compromise: inability to clear secretions, respiratory fatigue, poor oxygenation or ventilation
- Decreased level of consciousness where airway protective reflexes are impaired.
- Anticipated patient transfer of large burn with airway issue without qualified personnel to intubate en route

If bronchoscopy is performed, then consider the concurrent placement of an endotracheal tube (ETT) over the bronchoscope at the same time. Thereby reducing the number of airway manipulations. The ETT should be well secured for the transfer either with adhesive tape or umbilical tape passed around the back of the head.

If inhalation injury is suspected, then a carboxyhemoglobin level should be obtained and calculated back to the time of the burn injury. Carbon monoxide has a half-life of about 4 hours when breathing room air and around 1 hour when breathing 100% oxygen. A carboxyhemoglobin level of >60% has a >50% chance of mortality (**Box 1 and 2**).

Catabolism and Hypermetabolism

Burns covering large TBSA in children lead to an unprecedented hypermetabolic response that can last up to 2 years following initial injury. This response can be thought of as an exaggerated and protracted fright and flight reaction. The usual storm of cytokines, catecholamines, cortisol, and glucagon are released in massive quantities and for a sustained

Box 1 Carboxyhemoglobin (%) and symptoms	
Carboxyhemoglobin (%)	Symptoms
0–10	Normal
10–20	Headache, confusion
20–40	Disorientation, fatigue, nausea, visual changes
40–60	Hallucination, combativeness, convulsion, coma, shock state
60–70	Coma, convulsions, weak respiration and pulse
70–80	Decreasing respiration and stopping
80–90	Death in <1 h
90–100	Death within a few minutes

period. This period is characterized by a hyperdynamic cardiovascular response, increase in core body temperature, profoundly accelerated glycolysis, lipolysis, proteolysis, insulin resistance, liver dysfunction, and decreases of lean body mass and total body mass;[20–22] the result of which can lead to delayed wound healing and immune suppression.[23] Attenuation of this deleterious response can be achieved through both pharmacologic as well as non-pharmacological measures. Early enteral feeding, a warm environment, early excision and wound closure, meticulous infection control, and early exercise all contribute to combat the hypermetabolic response and maintain lean body mass.[24] Pharmacologic measures used to attenuate the catabolism resulting from the hypermetabolic

Box 2 Treatment for inhalation injury	
Treatment	Frequency
Turn side to side	q 2 h
Sitting or rocked in chair	As soon as physiologically stable
Ambulation	Early
Chest physiotherapy	q 2 h
Suctioning and lavage (nasal/oral tracheal)	q 2 h
Bronchodilators	q 2 h
Aerosolized heparin/ acetylcysteine	q 2 h alternating
Heparin 5000–10, 000 units with 3 mL normal saline	q 4 h
Alternated with acetylcysteine 20% 3 mL	q 4 h

response include propranolol, recombinant growth hormone, insulin, insulin-like growth factor-1, and anabolic steroids such as testosterone and oxandrolone.[21]

Early enteral nutrition not only gives the patient increased support during the hypermetabolic response but it also preserves gut mucosal integrity and improves intestinal blood flow and motility. Liquid enteral feeds are not required in small burns less than 10% TBSA, who should receive a high-protein, high-calorie diet alone. However, large burns above 30% TBSA would benefit from enteral feeds given either via nasoduodenal or nasojejunal feeding tubes.

Several formulas exist to calculate the nutritional requirements, in which the most popular are the Modified Curreri (utilizing basal metabolic rate [BMR]) and Galveston formulae:

Modified Curreri formula.
Infant: BMR + 15 kcal/%
Toddler: BMR + 25 kcal/%
Child: BMR + 40 kcal/%
7.
Galveston formula.
Infant: $2100 \text{ kcal/m}^2 + 1000 \text{ kcal/m}^2$ burn.
Child: $1800 \text{ kcal/m}^2 + 1300 \text{ kcal/m}^2$ burn.
Adolescent: $1500 \text{ kcal/m}^2 + 1500 \text{ kcal/m}^2$ burn.

Wound care

Early assessment of the burn wound by an experienced surgeon is essential to have the best outcome. Superficial partial-thickness injuries can be managed non-operatively and should heal within 10 to 14 days with dressing changes alone. Deep full-thickness injuries require early excision and grafting. It is occasionally difficult to determine the level of injury and differentiate between a partial thickness injury that will heal and a deep partial thickness injury that requires early excision and grafting, if unlikely to heal by 3 weeks (after which point the risk of hypertrophic scarring is significant).

Although topical antimicrobial agents were traditionally applied to partial-thickness injuries, the repeated dressing changes were found to be very painful and detracted from the use in children. Immediate application of silver-containing dressings at the time of cleaning has led to a reduction in frequency of dressing changes and hence associated pain.

Early excision and wound closure of large burns in children is both safe and effective in reducing sepsis, leading to a shorter length of hospital stay and reduced mortality.[25] The use of temporizing agents such as allograft, Biodegradable Temporizing Matrix (BTM), and Integra can all be used to close the wound until such time as sufficient donor

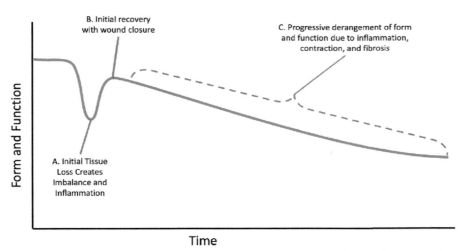

Fig. 1. Form and function deteriorate after initial recovery and acute wound closure due to ongoing inflammation and contraction in burn wounds.

site is available for autografting.[26] A drawback to autografting is leaving a visible scar at the donor site, which can cause problems of its own such as pruritis, pain and alterations in pigmentation, and sensation.[27] Therefore, the use of autologous engineered skin substitutes such as cultured epidermal autografts and other cell therapies[28–31] can be an effective to cover large burn wounds when donor sites are limited.

Pain Management and Psychological Care

Children recovering from large burn injuries will experience several different types of pain, each dealt with differently. Background pain which can usually be attenuated with acetaminophen or hydrocodone combinations, codeine, tramadol, and ibuprofen. Procedural pain, due to staple removal or major dressing changes, for which much stronger analgesia is required such as ketamine, together with an anxiolytic such as lorazepam. Finally, neuropathic pain resulting in burning sensations in the skin

Eriksonian Stages of Development

1. Trust or *Mistrust*
2. Autonomy or *Shame*
3. Initiative or *Guilt*
4. Industry or *Inferiority*
5. Identity or *Role Confusion*
6. Intimacy or *Isolation*
7. Generativity or *Stagnation*
8. Ego Integrity or *Despair*

Fig. 2. The Eriksonian model of development highlights alternate psychosocial outcomes for the growing child.

or phantom limb pain following amputation; this requires the use of gabapentin, pregabalin, or occasionally local anesthetic patches. Initial assessment of pain and anxiety can be carried out in children using a visual analogue scale, in order to gauge the success, or failure, of any intervention. In order to offset the gastrointestinal complications of this multimodal approach to pain, a bowel regimen must also be tailored to the individual.

With the ever-present risk of addiction, new strategies involving non-pharmacological distraction techniques (virtual reality and music therapy) have shown promising results with little to no reduction in effectiveness over time.[32]

Pediatric Burn Reconstruction

Dividing up the present article into an acute and reconstruction section raises the age-old question: what exactly is burn reconstruction and when does it start? In addition to the acute loss of tissue from the original burn, severe burns begin a process of inflammation, fibrosis, and contraction which deteriorates form and function as long as they continue (**Fig. 1**). This can include joint capsular contractures, joint subluxations, overall loss of range of motion, ectropions, and restraint of skeletal growth. When treatment is delayed, these sequelae can become difficult if not impossible to optimally correct. Hence, classic "reconstructive" interventions must take place whenever the ratio of Benefit/(Cost + Risk) indicates.

Creating the best possible long-term plan can be challenging in any severe burn. Adding considerations of growth and development renders this even more complex. Given cookie-cutter solutions do not work, we look more toward principles in

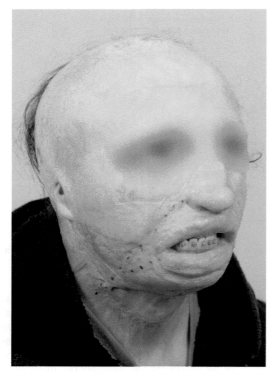

Fig. 3. Midfacial growth retardation due to severe burn.

developing a patient-specific plan. In the following text, the authors will review key principles of pediatric burn reconstruction which have stood the test of time in our hands.

Many enduring principles were famously described by Gillies and Millard[33] in the 1950s,

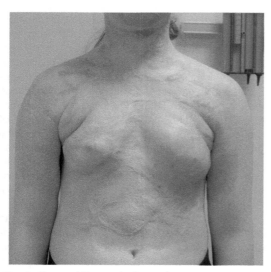

Fig. 4. Trapped Breast during puberty.

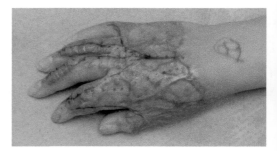

Fig. 5. A classic dorsal burn scar contracture following split thickness skin grafting.

arising from their experience as plastic surgeons in WWI and WWII. And although these were not written specifically for the pediatric burn population, most are relevant such as.[33]

- Seek insight into the patient's true desires.
- Return what is normal to normal position and retain it there.
- Tissue losses should be replaced in kind.

Indeed, modern burn reconstructive surgeons reading the "Old Masters" may be humbled to find their own practice not meeting the quality and sophistication of preceding generations.[33–35] In the following text, the authors will explore an overview of their current approach to pediatric burn reconstruction with an emphasis on some of the ruling principles.

Let your therapeutic planning be informed by an understanding of growth and development
Erik Erikson's well-known 8 stages of psychosocial development taught us that children are in the midst of a journey which may proceed to either full maturity or become tragically derailed[36] (Fig. 2). Burn injury and the care we provide can be dehumanizing pushing children in a direction of mistrust, inferiority, isolation, and despair.

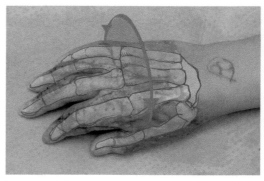

Fig. 6. Visualizing the anatomy and the full tissue deficit is the key.

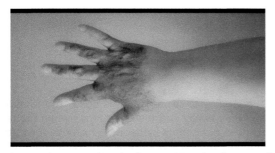

Fig. 7. The same hand after incisional release and addition of full-thickness skin grafts.

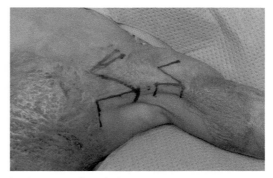

Fig. 9. Square flap designs.

Understanding that we need to proactively avoid psychosocial harm and promote healthy development in our approach to burn reconstruction is important. Pediatric burn reconstruction is therefore all about placing the child as quickly as possible back on track. Certainly, the relationship between the team and the patient/family should be one that is trustworthy, promotes autonomy, and empowers the patient, setting up for success with further development (see **Fig. 2**).

Physical and Intellectual Growth and Development

From a physical standpoint, proportions of much of the growing body are relatively stable over time with the important exception of the head and thighs. The infant has a large head and small thighs whereas the adult has large thighs and a proportionately smaller head. Examination of the Lund & Browder charts over time demonstrates that about age 5 leading up to the start of the pubertal growth spurt is the period where this transition happens. Other key landmarks in the growing child from a reconstructive perspective include the following.

Cranial vault growth is 85% complete by age 3

Brain and cranial growth are rapid in first 3 years of life plateauing at age 3. The reconstructive

consequence is that the scalp is an important source of skin when needed early.

Ear growth is stable at age 10

This also coincides with the time that costal cartilage becomes adequate for harvest total auricular construction via Nagata Technique.[37]

Pubertal Growth Velocity Peaks from Age 9 to 13

During this period, scars can become tighter with possible need for release or addition of tissue.

Skeletal and facial maturity occurs in the mid to late teens

Cicatricial restraint of facial dentoskeletal growth occurs classically following cleft palate repair. Severe facial cicatrix from burn can similarly restrain the sphenomaxillary suture posterior to the face creating an Angle Class III malocclusion and open bite. As in the case of cleft, final balancing via Le Fort I osteotomy and advancement should wait until the conclusion of facial growth with or without distraction depending on the severity of the scarring (**Fig. 3**).

For girls, breast development is complete by the 18 range

The breast bud is surprisingly resilient if not excised leading to breast development even with

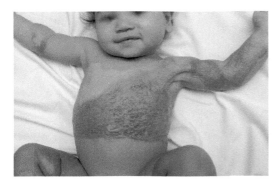

Fig. 8. Axillary contracture.

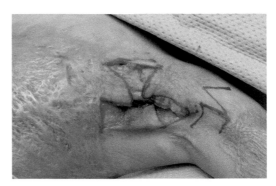

Fig. 10. Square flap after incision.

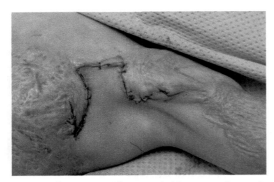

Fig. 11. After inset with normal skin across the entire scarred region.

a history of deep burn. Trapped breast symptoms of tightness and pain should be relieved as needed typically with incisional release and grafting as in **Fig. 4**. Final breast reconstruction may require adjustments in volume, shape, and cover ranging from implants, fat grafting, skin grafts, or flaps. The chronically constricted thorax should be treated with caution as incisional releases can yield larger wounds than anticipated and the scar can be relatively poorly perfused predisposing to wound healing problems and infections.

Other important landmarks that are ever in mind as surgical plans are developed include important intellectual and social ones such as.

- Early reading acquisition
- School integration
- Sports integration

Invest in and grow the therapeutic rapport/bank account

The journey to reintegration is costly to the child and their family and there are times when the resources are simply inadequate to move forward. One key resource upon which progress depends is the therapeutic rapport/bank account developed between the burn team and the patient and their family.

The therapeutic bank account is filled when patients/children experience wins in the therapeutic process, pain/anxiety/suffering is managed well, their agency/personhood is supported, and the team behaves in a trustworthy fashion. In contrast, breaches of trust, complications, incompetence, dishonesty, miscommunication, and the like empty the therapeutic bank account.

Children who are in an Eriksonian psychosocial disaster may be running on empty and not be good operative candidates until these issues are improved. Sometimes the authors' bank account with the patient/family is so low they offer surgery on borrowed trust. This is a relatively risky proposition but may be the first step out of a vicious circle for the patient. Some derivative principles along these lines include.

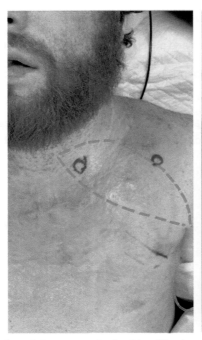
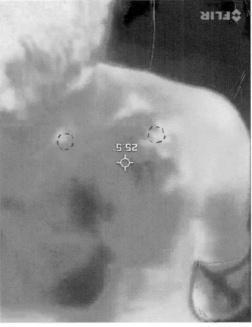

Fig. 12. Infrared thermography for identification and confirmation of perforators in burned tissue.

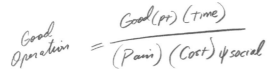

$$Good\ Operation = \frac{Good\ (pt)\ (time)}{(Pain)\ (Cost)\ \psi\ social}$$

Fig. 13. Equation for a good operation.

- Remember, every intervention draws upon the rapport/account you have built.
- Strive for speed and efficiency.
- Strive for a favorable cost-benefit balance for the child during every intervention.
- Minimize interruption of normal childhood.

Strive for accuracy in estimating the true magnitude of the tissue deficit

Less experienced surgeons perform z-plasties or other adjustments without understanding how much tissue is actually missing. Sterling Bunnell, the founder of modern hand surgery in the United States, stated the importance of this issue arising from his experience in the World Wars:

In contemplating repair of a contracted hand, we should first picture in our imagination the normal hand with a clear conception of its anatomy and physiology. Only then can we perceive and calculate the defects in skin and deeper structures, nerve, lymph and blood supply, muscle balance, and nutrition[35] (**Figs. 5–7**)

The reconstruction can only be as good as the release

This is another way of referring to Gillies' principle, "Return what is normal to normal position and retain it there."[33] But it is important to emphasize as the task of achieving a full release is often impeded by the following factors.

1. Fear of creating a defect the surgeon is not prepared to reconstruct.
2. Fear of injuring deep vital structures due to unfamiliarity with the anatomy
3. Failing to appreciate the big picture of the whole contracture.

Sufficed to say, we must all strive to be better than this.

All things being equal, seek to upgrade perfusion of any given reconstruction

Well vascularized tissues offer several distinct advantages when used in burn reconstruction.

1. The capacity to expand in response to tension.
2. Superior relief of tension due to #1.
3. Improved capacity to heal.
4. Improved resistance to infection.
5. The capacity to grow in children.

Figs. 8–11 demonstrate 1 common application of this in the pediatric axilla. A burn extending from the thorax across the anterior axilla into the medial arm will demand release. Incisional release and skin grafting is reserved only for the most severe pan-axillary contractures when no local options are available. Vascularized tissue in the form of local tissue rearrangement interrupts contracting scar with pliant vascularized tissue with the capacity to expand under tension as well as grow. This example demonstrates the "square flap" a favorite of Ogawa and Hyakusoku.[38]

Another tactic for upgrading vascularity of flaps in the authors' practice has been to identify and incorporate intact perforators when planning local flaps. Infrared thermography first introduced by Hallock and colleagues[39] with an inexpensive mobile phone attachment permits rapid scanning of a

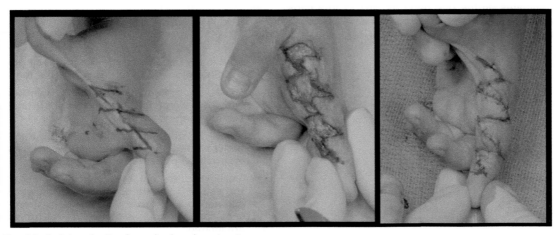

Fig. 14. Serial z-plasties for volar hand contracture.

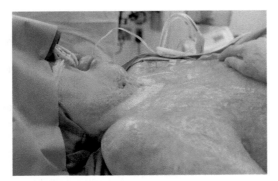

Fig. 15. Severe neck contracture.

large area for intact vessels. **Fig. 12** demonstrates the supraclavicular pedicle intact in a previously burned area in this case in anticipation of tissue expansion.

Strong Indicators for Surgery in Children

As previously indicated, every trip to the operation comes at a price for the child. But too much delay can permit deterioration of contractures and other issues. A good operation, as summarized in **Fig. 13** has a favorable ratio of good accomplished to the pain and psychosocial cost of intervention. One strong indication for intervention is persistent abnormal hand posture or joint subluxation due to scar. **Fig. 14** demonstrates a common volar contact burn in a toddler that has created a fixed flexion contracture in this case, amenable to serial z-plasties. Neck contractures can be extremely symptomatic particularly when they are involved in a larger complex that causes lip or eyelid ectropion. Those that prevent the patient from achieving a neutral gaze certainly require intervention. In the authors' practice, the authors favor full-thickness skin grafts although other options such as dermal templates on the one hand as well as free flaps on the other both have their place. **Figs. 15–17** demonstrate a severe neck contracture after a

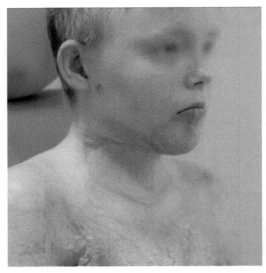

Fig. 17. Long-term result from full-thickness skin graft for the neck.

single release with platysmotomy and full-thickness skin grafting from the abdomen.

SUMMARY

As the authors have emphasized, the child with burn reconstructive needs is a bit of a moving target due to the active growth and development they are experiencing. Incorporating an understanding of developmental phases psychosocially and physically will pay dividends as the therapeutic team seeks to get the child through very difficult times. Fortunately, children are inherently resilient our work is one of the most rewarding endeavors imaginable in medicine.

CLINICS CARE POINTS

- Burn injury remains among the top 10 causes of unintentional injury and death in children.[1]
- Small burns should be irrigated for 20 minutes with cool water to diminish the depth and extent of injury.
- Delays in starting resuscitation of burned patients result in worse outcomes, this is especially important in children.
- Small children and especially those under the age of 1 should also receive a separate maintenance dextrose fluid solution to prevent hypoglycemia as their glycogen stores are limited.

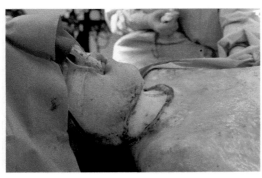

Fig. 16. Incisional release and full-thickness skin graft.

DISCLOSURE

The authors have nothing to disclose.

REFERENCES

1. Stewart S, Juang D, Aguayo P. Pediatric burn review. Semin Pediatr Surg 2022;31(5):151217.
2. Bull J, Fisher A. A study of mortality in a burns unit - a revised estimate. Ann Surg 1954;139(3):269–74.
3. Wolf S, Rose J, Desai M, et al. Mortality determinants in massive pediatric burns - an analysis of 103 children with >=80% TBSA burns (>=70% full-thickness). Ann Surg 1997;225(5):554–65.
4. Shah A, Liao L. Pediatric burn care unique considerations in management. Clin Plast Surg 2017;44(3):603–+.
5. Lee C, Mahendraraj K, Houng A, et al. Pediatric burns: a single institution retrospective review of incidence, etiology, and outcomes in 2273 burn patients (1995-2013). J Burn Care Res 2016;37(6):E579–85.
6. Cox S, Martinez R, Glick A, et al. A review of community management of paediatric burns. Burns 2015;41(8):1805–10.
7. Patel K, Rodríguez-Mercedes S, Grant G, et al. Physical, psychological, and social outcomes in pediatric burn survivors ages 5 to 18 Years: a systematic review. J Burn Care Res 2022;43(2):343–52.
8. Woolard A, Hill N, McQueen M, et al. The psychological impact of paediatric burn injuries: a systematic review. BMC Publ Health 2021;21(1):2281.
9. Kim L, Martin H, Holland A. Medical management of paediatric burn injuries: best practice. J Paediatr Child Health 2012;48(4):290–5.
10. Lu M, Zhao J, Wang X, et al. Research advances in prevention and treatment of burn wound deepening in early stage. Frontiers in Surgery 2022;9:1015411.
11. McAlister P, Hagan G, Lowry C, et al. Fifteen-minute consultation: management of paediatric minor burns. Archives of Disease in Childhood-Education and Practice Edition 2023;108(4):242–7.
12. Palmieri T. Pediatric burn resuscitation. Crit Care Clin 2016;32(4):547–+.
13. Datta PK, Roy Chowdhury S, Aravindan A, et al. Medical and surgical care of critical burn patients: a comprehensive review of current evidence and practice. Cureus 2022;14(11):e31550.
14. Mileder LP, Urlesberger B, Schwaberger B. Use of intraosseous vascular access during neonatal resuscitation at a tertiary center. Front Pediatr 2020;8:571285.
15. Scrivens A, Reynolds PR, Emery FE, et al. Use of intraosseous needles in neonates: a systematic review. Neonatology 2019;116(4):305–14.
16. Szarpak L, Ladny JR, Dabrowski M, et al. Comparison of 4 pediatric intraosseous access devices: a randomized simulation study. Pediatr Emerg Care 2020;36(10):e568–72.
17. Stevens JV, Prieto NS, Ridelman E, et al. Weight-based vs body surface area-based fluid resuscitation predictions in pediatric burn patients. Burns 2023;49(1):120–8.
18. Carvajal HF. Fluid resuscitation of pediatric burn victims: a critical appraisal. Pediatr Nephrol 1994;8(3):357–66.
19. Carvajal HF. A physiologic approach to fluid therapy in severely burned children. Surg Gynecol Obstet 1980;150(3):379–84.
20. Berger MM, Pantet O. Nutrition in burn injury: any recent changes? Curr Opin Crit Care 2016;22(4):285–91.
21. D'Cruz R, Martin HC, Holland AJ. Medical management of paediatric burn injuries: best practice part 2. J Paediatr Child Health 2013;49(9):E397–404.
22. Korkmaz HI, Flokstra G, Waasdorp M, et al. The complexity of the post-burn immune response: an overview of the associated local and systemic complications. Cells 2023;12(3):345.
23. Zhang M, Yang P, Yu T, et al. Lytic cocktail: an effective method to alleviate severe burn induced hypermetabolism through regulating white adipose tissue browning. Heliyon 2022;8(3):e09128.
24. Romanowski KS, Palmieri TL. Pediatric burn resuscitation: past, present, and future. Burns Trauma 2017;5:26.
25. Herndon DN, Parks DH. Comparison of serial debridement and autografting and early massive excision with cadaver skin overlay in the treatment of large burns in children. J Trauma 1986;26(2):149–52.
26. Palackic A, Duggan RP, Campbell MS, et al. The role of skin substitutes in acute burn and reconstructive burn surgery: an updated comprehensive review. Semin Plast Surg 2022;36(1):33–42.
27. Palmieri TL. Emerging therapies for full-thickness skin regeneration. J Burn Care Res 2023;44(Suppl_1):S65–7.
28. Hickerson WL, Remmers AE, Recker DP. Twenty-five years' experience and beyond with cultured epidermal autografts for coverage of large burn wounds in adult and pediatric patients, 1989-2015. J Burn Care Res 2019;40(2):157–65.
29. Lee H. Outcomes of sprayed cultured epithelial autografts for full-thickness wounds: a single-centre experience. Burns 2012;38(6):931–6.
30. Leclerc T, Thepenier C, Jault P, et al. Cell therapy of burns. Cell Prolif 2011;44(Suppl 1):48–54.
31. Jorgensen AM, Mahajan N, Atala A, et al. Advances in skin tissue engineering and regenerative medicine. J Burn Care Res 2023;44(Suppl_1):S33–41.
32. Hoffman HG, Chambers GT, Meyer WJ, et al. Virtual reality as an adjunctive non-pharmacologic analgesic for acute burn pain during medical procedures. Ann Behav Med 2011;41(2):183–91.

33. Gillies HdSaM, Magill I, Millard DR. The Principles and Art of Plastic Surgery Chapter on Anaesthesia by Ivan Magill, etc. London; printed in U.S.A. London, UK: Butterworth & Co; 1957.

34. Tolhurst D, SpringerLink (online service). Pioneers in plastic surgery: Available at: https://link.springer.com/book/10.1007/978-3-319-19539-1. Accessed January 12, 2024.

35. Bunnell S, Howard LD. Surgery of the hand. Fourth impression. Philadelphia, London, Montreal: J. B. Lippincott Company; 1944.

36. Erikson EH. Childhood and society. London: Imago Pub; 1950.

37. Nagata S. A new method of total reconstruction of the auricle for microtia. Plast Reconstr Surg 1993; 92(2):187–201.

38. Hyakusoku H, Fumiiri M. The square flap method. Br J Plast Surg 1987;40(1):40–6.

39. Hallock GG. Smartphone thermal imaging can enable the safer use of propeller flaps. Semin Plast Surg 2020;34(3):161–4.

Head and Neck Reconstruction in Burn Patients

Rei Ogawa, MD, PhD, FACS

KEYWORDS

• Thin flap • Skin pedicled flap • Skin graft • Perforator flap • Supercharging • Expanded flap

KEY POINTS

• In head and neck reconstruction, it is crucial to sufficiently relieve the tension on the neck.
• If using a skin flap, the skin-pedicled flap releases contracture more effectively than the island flap.
• During planning, it is necessary to consider the gender of the patient gender and the timing of the reconstruction.
• It is beneficial to use a large and thin single flap, preferably one whose vasculature can be supercharged.

INTRODUCTION

Reconstruction of burns in the head and neck area is particularly challenging because there is a high demand for both functional reconstruction that restores the complex movements of the neck and esthetic reconstruction. Local flaps are best for minor defects, especially deep burns, because their texture and color match. However, for large deep burn wounds that have led to scar contractures, it is crucial to ensure that the contractures are fully released and re-contracture will not occur. In this case, simple skin grafting or local flaps often do not yield satisfactory results.

According to data on Asians, the average skin thickness (including the epidermis and dermis) varies markedly depending on the body region.[1] Thus, the skin thicknesses on the cheek, chin, anterior neck, upper clavicle, and anterior chest are 1140, 860, 1410, 770, and 1440 μm, respectively[1] (**Table 1**). The areas where bones are located directly under the skin (ie, the chin and upper clavicle) tend to have thin skin. This means that reconstructing these areas with a thick flap will not provide esthetic results. Rather, their contour should be carefully reproduced by either using thin flaps or thick skin grafts. However, with regard

to full-thickness skin grafts, it is difficult to reconstruct a large skin defect that runs from the jaw to the chest with them. Moreover, skin grafts in highly mobile areas such as the neck may not sufficiently prevent secondary scar contracture because they lack a fatty layer. It should be noted that there is 1 exception to this, namely, the face; although the face is highly mobile, skin grafts are the primary choice for facial defects since they often successfully reconstruct burn wounds in the peri-oral and peri-orbital areas. Thus, extensive deep burns of the neck are best reconstructed with a large thin flap, since they yield excellent results.[2] In this article, the author will discuss the usefulness of thin flaps for reconstructing head and particularly neck burns, since the latter are highly prone to burn scar contracture.

INDICATION FOR RECONSTRUCTION

To identify the optimal approach to face and neck reconstruction, it is important to first classify the defects in the chin-neck-anterior chest units in terms of their size and depth[3] (**Box 1**). Wound depth can be broadly categorized as superficial to the platysma or deeper than the platysma; in the case of the neck, this means the wound does

Department of Plastic, Reconstructive and Aesthetic Surgery, Nippon Medical School, 1-1-5 Sendagi, Bunkyo-ku, Tokyo 113-0022, Japan
E-mail address: r.ogawa@nms.ac.jp

Clin Plastic Surg 51 (2024) 391–398
https://doi.org/10.1016/j.cps.2024.02.003

Table 1
Differences in skin thickness, as determined by cadaver study in Asian men and women

	Male (μm)	Female (μm)
Cheek	1240	1040
Chin	890	750
Anterior neck	1560	1260
Supraclavicular	960	560
Anterior chest	1390	1490
Abdomen	1440	1230
Back	2280	1470
Inguinal	500	500
Anterior thigh	1160	1080

The data show the average skin (epidermis and dermis) thickness of Asian men and women.

or does not reach the sternocleidomastoid muscle. Wound size is categorized as linear/planar scar contractures or small/large defects and whether the contracture/defect is confined within a unit or extends into adjacent units; in the case of the neck, its units encompass the central region and the left-right regions that are bounded by the sternocleidomastoid muscle.[3]

Linear scar contractures or small skin defects that are confined within a neck unit can be reconstructed with Z-plasty or various local flaps. However, if the linear scar contracture extends into an adjacent unit, it is necessary to release the contracture and ensure that the 2 units are clearly separated; this prevents re-contracture.

By contrast, planar scar contractures or extensive skin defects should be reconstructed with thick

Box 1
Classification of preoperative face and neck scar contractures for determining reconstruction options

I Linear scar contracture or small skin defects confined within each unit

II Linear scar contracture or small skin defects extending into adjacent units

III Planar scar contracture or large skin defects confined within each unit

IIIa Does not reach the muscle (in the neck, does not reach the sternocleidomastoid)

IIIb Reaches the muscle (in the neck, reaches the sternocleidomastoid)

IV Planar scar contracture or large skin defects extending into adjacent units

V Those that cannot be classified into I–IV

skin grafts or flaps. Depending on the case, an expander can also be used.[4] If the contractures or large skin defects remain within a single unit, the choice between a skin graft and flap depends on the depth of the reconstruction site. If it does not reach the platysma, a skin graft can be used. These grafts must be full thickness and their primary aim is to prevent (re)contracture and pigmentation. They can be combined with a dermal regeneration template such as Integra.[5] Thick skin grafts that preserve the subdermal vascular network (SVN)[6] can also be used but they will require reliable compression and fixation techniques.

For deep scar contractures or skin defects that reach an adjacent unit, or remain within 1 unit but reach the platysma, flaps are a good choice. It is desirable to use a large thin flap whose color and texture closely matches that of the neck.[7] To select the optimal flap, it is necessary to determine the range of reconstruction needed and the available donor sites.

TENSION RELEASE

The head and neck primarily extend and flex significantly in the anteroposterior direction. This means that chin-neck-anterior chest burns frequently develop into pathologic scars such as hypertrophic scars and keloids; these are abnormal skin fibroses that arise after skin injuries, especially burns, and can lead to scar contractures. Skin tension is a major risk factor for the formation of these scars.[8] Thus, a key objective when reconstructing burn defects, including contractures, in chin-neck-anterior chest region is to relieve tension in the anteroposterior direction. Flaps are particularly useful for releasing or preventing contracture because flaps bearing subcutaneous tissues expand naturally after surgery; this means that they are not prone to postsurgical hypertrophic scarring or contractures. By contrast, skin grafts do not expand. This means that skin grafts are stiff and cannot release the repetitive skin tension induced by daily movements of the neck and upper limbs. As a result, skin grafts tend to generate circular scars around the grafted skin that often progress into secondary contractures (**Fig. 1**). This link between skin stiffness and contractures also explain why burn scars, which are very stiff, are prone to forming contractures on the neck (and other mobile areas).

Thus, flaps are particularly useful for reconstructing the head and neck region. Ideally, these flaps should have skin pedicles because they expand better than island flaps and therefore release contractures more effectively[9] (**Fig. 2**). Moreover, the postoperative extensibility of the

Burned scars   Grafted skin

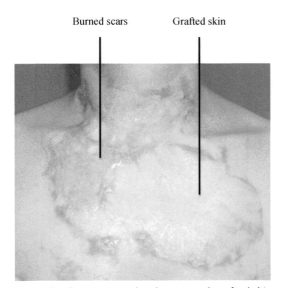

Fig. 1. Circular scars can develop around grafted skin. Since grafted skin and the scars on the margin of the graft are stiff, the skin tension produced by body movements such as turning of the head cannot be released. This causes the margin of graft to become inflamed and generates hypertrophic scars or keloids. Since these scars themselves are very stiff, they can readily progress into contractures.

flap should be considered when determining the optimal flap design for the individual patient. If the area of reconstruction is large, large local flaps with supercharged vessels can be designed.[10] If adjacent skin cannot be used as a flap-donor site, free flaps should be selected. However, this is the least preferred choice because free flaps are always island flaps; thus, they will not expand effectively and may be prone to hypertrophic scarring/secondary contractures. Thus, for deep scar contractures, the order of choice should be (1) a skin-pedicled local flap/supercharged skin-pedicled flap and (2) a free flap.

TIMING OF RECONSTRUCTION

Large burns and their resulting extensive wound-healing process provoke a prolonged systemic cytokine storm.[11] This may be a major risk factor for the formation of hypertrophic scars and keloids after burn. This notion is supported by recent studies that suggest these pathologic scars can be promoted by systemic factors, including hypertension, female hormones, and high levels of various cytokines and growth factors in the blood.[11] Consequently, it is thought that reconstructive surgery within 1 year of sustaining a burn injury, particularly with poorly extensible skin grafts or local flaps, bears a high risk of

postoperative pathologic scarring and severe contracture. This risk may be even greater in cases with conditions such as hypertension. A potential way to minimize this risk is to use as much as possible single large thin flaps for reconstruction.

BASICS OF FLAP HARVESTING

A large thin skin flap is appropriate in cases IIIb and IV in **Box 1**, namely, if the neck scar reaches the sternocleidomastoid and is also a linear scar contracture/small unit-confined or unit-crossing defect/large unit-confined defect (IIIb) or a planar scar contracture/large unit-crossing defect (IV). Depending on the situation, one should choose either a vascular-pedicled flap or a free flap that has a vascular pedicle. An expander may also be utilized. If the burn is extensive, the number of donor sites that are available will be limited. However, the author will review here the hypothetical case where all donor sites are available. A number of points regarding flap harvest should be considered.

Skin Color and Texture

The upper-clavicular and anterior-chest regions are classical cases of areas that generally have 1 donor site available that can yield skin flaps that closely match the recipient site in terms of color and texture (**Fig. 3**). In this case, the donor site is the back; even if the case involves extensive burns, the skin of the back is often preserved. However, it should be noted that in males, the back skin is slightly thicker than the neck skin. Other donor-site possibilities are the abdomen, thigh, and inguinal regions. However, in Asian people, the abdomen and thigh regions are paler than the neck while the inguinal area tends to be darker. Moreover, the abdomen and inguinal areas have a different texture than the chin and anterior neck, which makes them challenging to use for reconstruction. However, bilateral inguinal flaps have been reported to have good outcomes when used for anterior neck reconstruction.

Gender Differences in Skin Thickness

Women and men differ in the skin thickness in various areas. Specifically, in Asian men and women, the anterior neck/back skin-thickness ratio is 1:1.5 and 1:1.2, respectively (see **Table 1**). Thus, harvesting a flap from the back and transplanting it to the anterior neck is generally more suitable for women (**Fig. 4**). Conversely, the anterior neck/chest ratio is 1:0.9 for men and 1:1.2 for women. Thus, chest-to-neck transplants are more suitable for men (**Fig. 5**) but not women. This is compounded

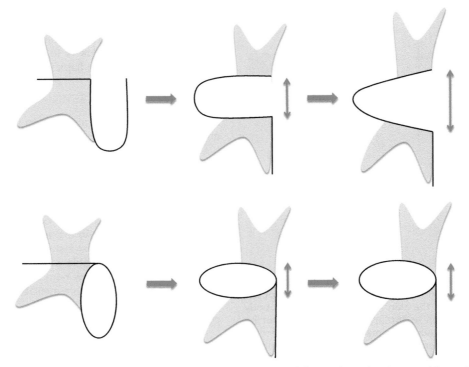

Fig. 2. Skin-pedicled flaps release tension much better than island flaps. Flaps that bear a skin pedicle (*top*) release the tension on the neck-anterior chest region that is induced by body movements. They also expand over time in the predominant direction of tension after surgery, thus further relieving the tension. By contrast, island flaps (bottom) expand poorly because of the lack of a skin pedicle. This makes these flaps prone to forming hypertrophic scars around their margin after surgery.

by the fact that harvesting flaps from the chest in women can result in asymmetrical breast positioning. Thus, for men, it is better to harvest from the chest, and for women, from the back. However, since the supraclavicular area is thin in both genders (less than 1000 μm), flaps from this region are suitable for reconstructing the chin and anterior neck in both men and women.

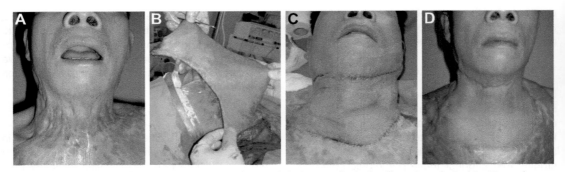

Fig. 3. Reconstruction of neck contracture with a pedicled supraclavicular flap. A male in his 40s underwent reconstruction of his anterior-neck contracture with a 25 × 15-cm supraclavicular flap. The flap was elevated as vascular-pedicled flap and survived completely. Although slight hypertrophic scars developed on the flap margin, the neck movement of the patient recovered to the point that he reported no problems in daily life. The donor site was closed by using a split-thickness skin graft. (*A*) Preoperative view. (*B*) Flap harvest. (*C*) Immediately after surgery. (*D*) One year after the operation. (With permission from the publisher: Vinh VQ, Van Anh T, Ogawa R, Hyakusoku H. Anatomical and clinical studies of the supraclavicular flap: analysis of 103 flaps used to reconstruct neck scar contractures. Plast Reconstr Surg. 2009 May;123(5):1471-1480.)

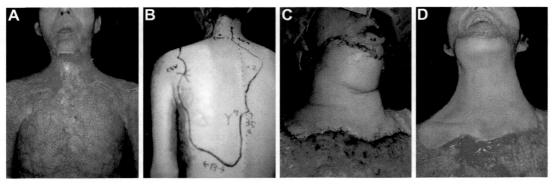

Fig. 4. Reconstruction of neck contracture with a flap from the back. A female in her 30s underwent reconstruction of her anterior-neck contracture with a large 35 × 19-cm skin-pedicled flap from the back. The circumflex scapular vessels and the seventh dorsal intercostal perforators (D-ICAPs) were attached to the flap and then anastomosed to the facial vessels and transverse cervical vessels, respectively. The flap survived fully and the contracture was effectively released. (A) Preoperative view. (B) Flap design. (C) Immediately after surgery. (D) Three weeks after surgery. (With permission from the publisher; Ogawa R, Hyakusoku H, Murakami M. Color Doppler ultrasonography in the planning of microvascular augmented "super-thin" flaps. Plast Reconstr Surg. 2003 Sep;112(3):822-8.)

Flap Thinness

The average skin thickness of the chin is 860 μm, whereas that of the anterior neck is 1410 μm.[1] In comparison, the supraclavicular area is very thin at 770 μm (see Table 1). Thus, the supraclavicular artery flap is an excellent choice when prioritizing flap thinness. Since the average skin thickness of the anterior chest and back is 1440 and 1980 μm, respectively, they can be used to reconstruct the 1410 μm-thick anterior-neck skin with minimal discomfort. However, these flaps are not suitable for reconstructing the 860 μm-thick chin skin because they can result in excessive thickness. Instead, very thin flaps such as super-thin flaps after primary fat-layer removal[7] or perforator flaps (discussed further in the following paragraphs)

should be used (see Fig. 4). Note also that after extensive burns, patients often lose weight. This can affect the thickness of the skin, meaning that thin flaps can often be harvested in burn patients without having to remove the fat. Conversely, as time progresses post-injury, the back and abdominal areas may accumulate fatty tissue, making the flaps thicker and necessitating fat removal. Patient weight loss and gain should be considered when selecting donor sites.

FLAP SELECTION
Pedicled Flaps

Flaps such as the pectoralis major, latissimus dorsi, and trapezius flaps can be pedicled and transplanted to the cervical region. However, due

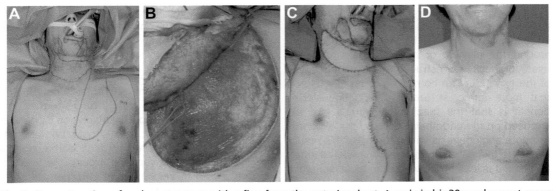

Fig. 5. Reconstruction of neck contracture with a flap from the anterior chest. A male in his 20s underwent reconstruction of his anterior-neck contracture with a large 22 × 7-cm skin-pedicled flap from the anterior chest. The second internal mammary artery perforator was attached to the flap and anastomosed to the facial artery and veins. The flap survived fully and the contracture was effectively released. (A) Preoperative view. (B) Flap harvest. (C) Immediately after surgery. (D) One and a half years after the operation.

to the thickness of these flaps, they may not be the top choices for reconstruction solely for scar contracture. Pedicled perforator flaps around the neck include the facial artery perforator,[12] superior thyroid artery perforator,[13] and transverse cervical artery perforator flaps[14] while the perforator flap in the shoulder area is the supraclavicular flap. Those in the chest include the internal thoracic artery perforator flap or internal mammary artery perforator flap[15] and the pectoral intercostal artery perforator flap,[16] while the superficial cervical artery perforator flap[17] has been reported to be available in the back.

Free Flaps

Essentially, all free flaps can be considered. However, the size, thickness, texture, color, and donor-site morbidity of the flap should be comprehensively assessed to determine suitability. Suitable free flaps for the neck include perforator flaps such as the thoracodorsal artery perforator flap[18] and the lateral thoracic artery perforator flap.[19]

Thinned Flaps

Thinned flaps are those that are nourished by the SVN and have had as much of the fat layer removed as possible. They have been termed SVN flaps,[20] super-thin flaps,[7] and microdissected flaps[21] but the most common terms internationally are super-thin and ultra-thin flaps. These flaps are known to be useful options for cervical scar-contracture reconstruction. The flaps that have been developed with thinning in mind[20] include the cervico-pectoral (CP) (see **Fig. 5**), occipito-CP, occipito-cervico-dorsal (see **Fig. 4**), and occipito-cervico-shoulder flaps.

Expanded Flaps

Expanders are especially suitable for children with limited donor skin or cases where cosmetic reconstruction is a priority.[22] Expanded flaps created around the clavicle or anterior chest are often used for neck reconstruction.[23] A disadvantage of the expander flap compared to regular flaps is that more surgeries are involved. However, a benefit is that the mechanical stimuli that are imposed on the endothelial cells by the expander promote angiogenesis within the flap. This results in a large thin flap that can be transplanted safely because it is less prone to postsurgical ischemia.

Prefabricated Flaps

While it seems that fewer prefabricated flaps are currently being used for cervical scar-contracture reconstruction, they may still be useful for simultaneous reconstruction of the beard with vascular bundle transplantation, or simultaneous reconstruction with deep tissues.[4] Prefabricated flaps may become useful again as tissue engineering technology progresses.

TIPS FOR HARVESTING THIN FLAPS SAFELY
Survival Area of Thin Skin Flaps

Numerous anatomic studies have been conducted to determine the maximal area of thin skin flaps (including perforator flaps) that will survive.[24] However, the survival area of thin skin flaps can vary depending on physiologic conditions such as blood pressure fluctuations. Thus, it is essential to design thin flaps with some margin, retain the skin pedicle to promote venous perfusion, and employ techniques such as supercharging to ensure the safe and consistent adherence of thin flaps. For example, a supercharged flap with 2 or more pedicles can be generated from a large thin flap harvested from the chest or back by adding perforators to the periphery of the flap and anastomosing them to the recipient site. Currently, flap survival area is estimated by preoperatively evaluating the internal vessels of the flap by multidetector computed tomography (MDCT).[25] However, further research on the safe survival area of thin flaps is needed.

Presence or Absence of Recipient Vessels

Before surgery, the patency of recipient vessels should be confirmed by methods such as MDCT, color Doppler, or sound Doppler.[7] In cases where there is a risk of poor vascular anastomosis, single vascular pedicle flaps will not be options. Moreover, thin flaps may have weak venous return, so if it is possible to use 2 or more perforators, harvesting one as a skin pedicle can stabilize the blood flow of the flap. This often achieves sufficient venous perfusion, even if the skin pedicle is narrow.

Defatting Procedure

Since the skin of the chin and anterior neck is thin, a defatting procedure should be performed in a single stage before flap transplantation if possible. During this process, care should be taken to remove the fatty layer without damaging the SVN. Thus, the fat removal around the vascular stem should be minimal, and for other parts, the fat should be removed to the point where the SVN is visible, leaving the least amount of fatty layer.[20] If a skin pedicle can be retained in the flap, it is safe to aggressively remove its fat because not only does the removal of this excess fat not affect the adherence of the flap, it can actually expand its adherence area.

SUMMARY

Since the head and neck primarily extend and flex significantly in the anteroposterior direction, a key point is how to relieve tension in this direction. It is crucial to assess the extent and depth of reconstruction that is needed throughout the face-neck-anterior chest region, and to make the choice between techniques such as Z-plasty, skin grafting, super-thin flaps, and free flaps, including perforator flaps, on the basis of the principles outlined in this article.

CLINICS CARE POINTS

- Tension sustains scar inflammation and increases the risk of hypertrophic scars and scar contracture.
- In head and neck reconstruction, the first priority is to release tension when selecting a flap.
- Skin pedicled flaps are more effective than island flaps in releasing tension, so they should be the first choice.
- For large flaps, supercharging the perforator branches can stabilize the blood flow.

DISCLOSURE

There are no conflict of interests.

REFERENCES

1. Lee Y, Hwang K. Skin thickness of Korean adults. Surg Radiol Anat 2002;24:183–9.
2. Orgill DP, Ogawa R. Current methods of burn reconstruction. Plast Reconstr Surg 2013;131(5): 827e–36e.
3. Ogawa R, Pribaz JJ. Diagnosis, assessment, and Classification of scar contractures. In: Hyakusoku H, Orgill DP, Teot L, et al, editors. Atlas of burn reconstructive surgery. Berlin-Heidelberg: Springer; 2010. p. 44–61.
4. Pribaz JJ, Fine N, Orgill DP. Flap prefabrication in the head and neck: a 10-year experience. Plast Reconstr Surg 1999;103(3):808–20.
5. Frame JD, Still J, Lakhel-LeCoadou A, et al. Use of dermal regeneration template in contracture release procedures: a multicenter evaluation. Plast Reconstr Surg 2004;113(5):1330–8.
6. Tsukada S. Transfer of free skin grafts with a preserved subcutaneous vascular network. Ann Plast Surg 1980;4(6):500–6.
7. Ogawa R, Hyakusoku H, Murakami M. Color Doppler ultrasonography in the planning of microvascular augmented "super-thin" flaps. Plast Reconstr Surg 2003;112(3):822–8.
8. Ogawa R. Mechanobiology of scarring. Wound Repair Regen 2011;19(Suppl 1):s2–9.
9. Yoshino Y, Kubomura K, Ueda H, et al. Extension of flaps associated with burn scar reconstruction: a key difference between island and skin-pedicled flaps. Burns 2018;44(3):683–91.
10. Hyakusoku H, Pennington DG, Gao JH. Microvascular augmentation of the super-thin occipito-cervico-dorsal flap. Br J Plast Surg 1994;47(7): 465–9.
11. Ogawa R. Keloid and hypertrophic scars are the result of Chronic Inflammation in the Reticular dermis. Int J Mol Sci 2017;18(3):606.
12. Horta R, Barreiro D, Nascimento R, et al. The facial artery perforator flap as a New option for reconstruction of Intraoral defects: Surgical Tips and clinical series. J Craniofac Surg 2019;30(5):1525–8.
13. Wilson JL, Rozen WM, Ross R, et al. The superior thyroid artery perforator flap: anatomical study and clinical series. Plast Reconstr Surg 2012;129(3): 641–6.
14. Chin T, Ogawa R, Murakami M, et al. An anatomical study and clinical cases of 'super-thin flaps' with transverse cervical perforator. Br J Plast Surg 2005;58(4):550–5.
15. Yu BT, Hsieh CH, Feng GM, et al. Clinical application of the internal mammary artery perforator flap in head and neck reconstruction. Plast Reconstr Surg 2013;131(4):520e–6e.
16. Oki K, Murakami M, Tanuma K, et al. Anatomical study of pectoral intercostal perforators and clinical study of the pectoral intercostal perforator flap for hand reconstruction. Plast Reconstr Surg 2009; 123(6):1789–800.
17. Ogawa R, Murakami M, Vinh VQ, et al. Clinical and anatomical study of superficial cervical artery flaps: retrospective study of reconstructions with 41 flaps and the feasibility of harvesting them as perforator flaps. Plast Reconstr Surg 2006;118(1): 95–101.
18. Mun GH, Jeon BJ, Lim SY, et al. Reconstruction of postburn neck contractures using free thin thoracodorsal artery perforator flaps with cervicoplasty. Plast Reconstr Surg 2007;120(6):1524–32.
19. Baghaki S, Cevirme M, Diyarbakirli M, et al. Locoregional use of lateral thoracic artery perforator flap as a propeller flap. Ann Plast Surg 2015;74(5):532–5.
20. Hyakusoku H, Gao JH, Pennington DG, et al. The microvascular augmented subdermal vascular network (ma-SVN) flap: its variations and recent

development in using intercostal perforators. Br J Plast Surg 2002;55(5):402–11.

21. Kimura N, Satoh K, Hosaka Y. Microdissected thin perforator flaps: 46 cases. Plast Reconstr Surg 2003;112(7):1875–85.

22. De La Cruz Monroy MFI, Kalaskar DM, Rauf KG. Tissue expansion reconstruction of head and neck burn injuries in paediatric patients - a systematic review. JPRAS Open 2018;18:78–97.

23. Gao JH, Ogawa R, Hyakusoku H, et al. Reconstruction of the face and neck scar contractures using staged transfer of expanded "Super-thin flaps". Burns 2007;33(6):760–3.

24. Karakawa R, Yoshimatsu H, Tanakura K, et al. An anatomical study of the lymph-collecting vessels of the medial thigh and clinical applications of lymphatic vessels preserving profunda femoris artery perforator (LpPAP) flap using pre- and intraoperative indocyanine green (ICG) lymphography. J Plast Reconstr Aesthet Surg 2020;73(9):1768–74.

25. Ono S, Hyakusoku H, Ogawa R, et al. Usefulness of multidetector-row computed tomography in the planning and postoperative assessment of perforator flaps. J Nippon Med Sch 2008;75(1):50–2.

The Role of Microsurgery in Burn Surgery

Mario Alessandri Bonetti, MD[a], Francesco M. Egro, MD, MSc, MRCS[a,b,*]

KEYWORDS

- Burns • Microsurgery • Prelaminated flaps • Prelamination • Prefabricated flaps • Prefabrication
- Burn reconstruction • Tissue engineering

KEY POINTS

- Microsurgical reconstruction in patients with burn is seldom the primary approach due to the clinical status of patients with burn, prolonged surgery, postoperative care demands, and the need for specialized training. Free flaps in acute burns exhibit a higher failure rate (approximately 10%), likely linked to the hyperinflammatory and hypercoagulable state of the severe burn patient. Strategies to improve outcomes include preoperative clinical status and nutrition optimization, careful anticoagulation, and considering timing and burn etiology in reconstruction planning.
- Burn contractures can severely impact range of motion and functional outcomes, affecting daily activities and overall well-being. Delayed burn reconstruction focuses on functional and aesthetic restoration, with free flaps being a primary choice for extensive contractures whereby local options are inadequate. Unlike in acute burns, elective reconstructive procedures show a comparable, low rate of flap loss. Additionally, free flaps reduce the risk of contracture recurrence by providing abundant, well-vascularized tissue that supports proper wound healing and minimizes tension on the scar. However, thorough removal of contracted tissue and addressing underlying structures are crucial to prevent persistent contractures and functional limitations.
- Prefabricated and prelaminated flaps have proven as effective reconstructive options in challenging facial burn reconstructions, showing optimal functional and aesthetic results. Despite the intricate nature of these cases, which often necessitate multiple surgeries, including revision and debulking procedures, prefabricated and prelaminated flaps prove to be able to dramatically improve burn survivors quality of life.

BACKGROUND

Burn injuries represent a worldwide health problem, registering over 8 million incidents globally in 2019.[1] Acute and reconstructive burns are a great challenge. Over the years, skin grafting has remained the mainstay treatment for acute partial and full-thickness burns, allowing coverage of large defects with minimal donor site morbidity. In cases whereby wounds are not amenable to immediate skin grafting, the temporary use of innovative technologies such as skin substitutes or negative pressure dressings can be chosen as bridge therapies between injury and reconstruction of acute burn injuries.[2,3] These approaches foster the formation of granulation tissue and neovascularization, frequently allowing for later skin grafting through a two-step approach. Nevertheless, when critical structures such as bones, cartilage, tendons, or neurovascular bundles are extensively exposed, opting for the flap reconstruction often emerges as the more suitable and appropriate strategy by granting a more robust and reliable coverage.[4–6] Flaps allow one-stage coverage of complex defects, shortening the healing time and reducing the risk of complications

[a] Department of Plastic Surgery, University of Pittsburgh Medical Center, Pittsburgh, PA, USA; [b] Department of Surgery, University of Pittsburgh Medical Center, Pittsburgh, PA, USA
* Corresponding author. Department of Plastic Surgery, University of Pittsburgh Medical Center, 1350 Locust Street, Medical Professional Building, Suite G103, Pittsburgh, PA 15219.
E-mail address: francescoegro@gmail.com

Clin Plastic Surg 51 (2024) 399–408
https://doi.org/10.1016/j.cps.2024.02.005
0094-1298/24/© 2024 Elsevier Inc. All rights reserved.

related to delayed wound healing, such as the dehydration and infection of the exposed structures. In circumstances whereby local flaps are unavailable or deemed unsuitable according to the extent of the injury, defect size and site, free tissue transfer remains the only option. Free flaps allow for the transfer of healthy and well-vascularized tissue from donor areas distant from the zone of injury, and allow for the coverage of deep and large defects in both acute and delayed burn reconstruction settings.

ACUTE BURN RECONSTRUCTION

Burn injuries lead to various anatomic and physiologic alterations in the body. They cause local and systemic responses due to the release of inflammatory mediators, potentially leading to organ dysfunction in more severe and extensive cases.[7] Key improvements in resuscitation and infection control have allowed a shift in focus toward more aggressive reconstructive plans for these challenging patients with acute burn.[7]

Reconstruction following an acute burn is generally classified as acute when carried out within 6 weeks from the day of injury.[8,9]

Burn injuries necessitating wound coverage are primarily managed with the use of skin grafts, which can cover a large surface area, particularly if meshed. Flap reconstruction is rarely required, with the usage of free flaps being even rarer. Perrault and colleagues queried the Nationwide Inpatient Sample database and found that out of 306,923 patients with acute burn, only 0.17% required a flap reconstruction (pedicled or free).[10] Following the principle of the reconstructive ladder, free flaps are reserved for severe and/or extensive wounds involving the exposure of critical structures (eg, bone, joints, tendons, and neurovascular structures) when local options are inadequate.[6,11-13]

Among the reasons why microsurgical reconstruction is seldom chosen as the primary approach for patients with acute burn there is the inherently prolonged nature of the surgery, which can be challenging for severely burned patients who often present with an unstable clinical status due to the systemic inflammatory sprout. Moreover, the postoperative period after a free flap procedure demands meticulous care and strict patient compliance, which may be difficult to achieve in patients with a wavering clinical condition. Furthermore, the intricate techniques involved in performing a free flap require specialized training; not every burn service may have access to a surgeon skilled enough to perform microsurgery. Lastly, despite the advancements in the knowledge

of the anatomy and physiology of free flaps, they still exhibit a variable, yet high, failure rate in patients with acute burn, further discouraging their use in this patient population. Among the largest series of free flap reconstruction in patients with acute burn, Baumeister and colleagues[8] reported a 23% rate of free flap failure in 43 patients. Shen and colleagues[14] counted a 13% failure rate in 49 patients undergoing 54 microsurgical flaps. Conversely, Pan and colleagues showed no failures in a cohort of 38 patients undergoing the microsurgical reconstruction of acute burn injuries of the upper extremity.[15] Our group recently performed a systematic review and meta-analysis showing a free flap failure rate of 10% in acute burns, with more than 20% of free flaps requiring revision and acute return to the operating room.[16] Therefore, the rate of free flap loss in acute burns appears to be much higher than the traditionally quoted free flap loss rate (between 2% and 5%) reported in other populations, such as patients undergoing elective postoncological reconstruction.[17,18] For these reasons, free flaps in the acute setting should be considered only if the wounds are not amenable to skin substitutes, skin grafts, or local flaps.

Despite the limited evidence is still available to shed light on the factors determining a higher flap loss rate in acute burns different mechanisms likely come into play, such as the local and systemic hyperinflammatory states that follow burn injuries. Such injuries increase vascular permeability and disrupt vascular integrity, leading to enhanced interstitial pressure and edema. The resulting edema can exert compressive forces, potentially hindering venous outflow. Moreover, the trauma and inflammation induce perivascular scarring, which may reduce the pliability of vessels, compromising both arterial inflow and venous outflow, and promote thrombi formation.[19] Burn injuries also cause endothelial damage and impair the contractility of perivascular smooth muscles. This damage, as observed by DeSpain et al.,[20] can lead to increased extracellular matrix protein expression, suggesting compromised vasodilation capacity. These processes combined with the significant inflammatory response determine a hypercoagulable state in patients with burn.[21] Research indicates that this hypercoagulability emerges 24 to 48 hours postburn and peaks around 2 to 3 weeks.[22,23] Consequently, this combination of a hypercoagulable state and endothelial damage may elevate the risk of arterial and venous thrombosis at the microvascular anastomosis site, explaining the observed high incidence of free flap failures in acute burns.

Despite still limited to clinical experience, several strategies may be used to improve surgical outcomes. Preoperative considerations include the need for preoperative clinical and nutrition optimization, and nerve blocks to reduce the vasospasm. Patients need to be off organ support including pressors and renal replacement therapy. Nutrition status needs to be monitored closely and it should be optimized by means of protein and vitamin supplementation. Edema should be optimized by wrapping and elevating the extremity. The authors have a very low threshold to start tube feeds if the patient is unable to maintain optimal nutrition by oral means. Good communication with the critical care, nutrition team, and anesthesia and regional anesthesia team are essential for planning and ensuring the patient is ready and safe to proceed with surgery. Careful consideration for intraoperative and postoperative anticoagulation is needed both during the anastomosis procedure and in the postoperative stage. Patients are routinely anticoagulated at the time of anastomosis and postoperatively. At the time of anastomosis, a 5000 units bolus of intravenous heparin is given. Postoperatively the following protocol is used: intravenous heparin at a rate of 500 units per hour, aspirin at 325 mg per rectum at the end of surgery followed by daily 81 mg, use of sequential compressive devices while in bed, bair hugger and warm room temperature, and early mobilization based on the location of the flap. Secondly, optimizing venous outflow and arterial inflow can be achieved through various maneuvers including performing the anastomosis outside the zone of injury, adventitial stripping, end-to-end anastomosis, 2 venous anastomoses, avoiding very large flaps, which might have higher requirements and the potential of partial necrosis, avoiding pedicle kinking, and prevent pedicle exposure, which is often challenging due to the absence of available viable soft tissue coverage.

Further understanding of the processes involved in acute burn injuries can contribute to the optimization of surgical strategies, aiming to reduce the risk of complications such as flap loss. For instance, the timing of the reconstruction is likely to play a pivotal role. Baumeister and colleagues[8] observed that the highest risk of flap failure occurred between day 5 and day 21 postinjury (8 out of 10 losses). This finding echoes the results reported by Pessoa Vaz and colleagues,[24] who experienced a 13% flap loss rate with all failures falling between day 5 and day 21 postinjury. Similarly, Pedrazzi and colleagues[25] documented a 17% flap failure rate, again with all losses confined to the same time window. The authors of this article conducted a systematic review and meta-analysis of 17 articles and 275 free flaps performed on 260 patients with acute burn. The study showed that the pooled prevalence of free flap failure was higher between 5 and 21 days from the day of injury (16.55%), or during the first 4 days (7.32%); however, the free flap failure rate was lowest after day 21 (6.74%).[26] Since the timing of the reconstruction appears to influence surgical outcomes, the senior author routinely delays free flap reconstruction until day 22 from the day of injury to reduce risk of flap loss.[26]

The role of the burn etiology and location are other factors under scrutiny. However, no definitive conclusion can still be drawn about their impact on the free flap failure rate. Perrault and colleagues[10] reported a significantly higher risk of flap loss in case of electrical burns compared with thermal. However, they included in the analysis any type of flap and not free flaps only. Baumeister and colleagues[8] found that flaps used for coverage of burns to the lower extremities had twice the failure rate compared with the upper extremities (21% vs 10%). Moreover, studies reporting lower rates of flap loss include patients with defects predominantly involving the upper extremity.[4,5] However, further studies are needed to confirm these findings. A summary of preoperative, intraoperative, and postoperative considerations can be found in **Table 1**.

Patient selection is critical to ensure optimal outcomes of patients (**Figs. 1** and **2**). Since microsurgical reconstruction may be the only alternative in limb salvaging situations, continued investigation into strategies to reduce the risk of free flap failure in acute burn is needed. This could ultimately result in better care and an enhanced quality of life for these patients.

DELAYED BURN RECONSTRUCTION

Advances in burn care over the years have reduced complications and mortality, increasing the importance of the quality of life and functionality of burn survivors.[27] Indeed, despite the developments in the acute management of burns, patients develop hypertrophic scars and contractures.[28] These contractures can then in turn have a great impact in the patient's life including decrease in range of motion, compromised functional outcomes.[29] The head and neck, as well as the upper/lower extremities are regions of high functional demand for fine and wide movements.[29] Impairment in the range of motion due to scar contracture and fibrosis results in an inability to perform everyday activities, impacting patients' physical well-being and overall quality of life.[30,31] The depth of the burn and the healing time directly correlate to the amount of scarring and the chance of developing a hypertrophic scar.[32-34] Various

Table 1
Preoperative, intraoperative and postoperative considerations in patients with acute burn requiring microsurgical reconstruction

Preoperative	Intraoperative	Postoperative
• Wait until day 21 from burn injury • TEG • Nutrition optimization • Edema optimization • Off organ support • Nerve blocks if reconstructing extremity	• Anastomosis outside of zone of injury when possible • Adventitial stripping • End-to-end anastomosis • Two vein anastomosis • Avoid pedicle kinking • Avoid pedicle exposure • Anticoagulation	• Anticoagulation • Maintain warm environment • Limb elevation

methods such as compression garments, massage, laser therapy, intense pulsed light, steroids, exercise, and fat grafting have been used to minimize hypertrophic scarring.[35] Despite providing benefits, these treatments alone may not be sufficient due to the evolving nature of burn scars and recurrence of contractures. Therefore, recurrent rounds of laser therapy, contracture release, and/or adjacent tissue transfer are generally needed.

Delayed burn reconstruction is performed on patients that have already received definitive acute burn surgical care and it aims at functional restoration by release of the contractures limiting the movement, at aesthetic and psychological improvement by reconstructing areas causing disfigurement by removing hypertrophic scars which are often raised, pigmented and cosmetically unpleasing; at pain and discomfort alleviation, by rearranging the scar tissue, which can cause pain, itching, and altered sensation.[36]

Free flaps are primarily used in burn delayed reconstruction in case extensive areas are involved in the contracture and no local option is deemed suitable for coverage of the soft tissue defect resulting after scar tissue excision.[37]

Contrary to the risk of flap loss seen in acute burns, patients undergoing reconstructive procedures are elective and seem to have a flap loss rate comparable to that in other elective patient populations. Among the largest studies available on the outcomes of free flap burn reconstruction, Angrigiani and colleagues[38] reported a rate of flap loss at 5.6% in 150 patients. De Lorenzi and colleagues[39] experienced 5.7% failure rate in 53 patients. Similarly, Ohkubo and colleagues[40] reported a flap loss rate of 5% in 99 patients undergoing free flap delayed burn reconstruction. In addition, many recent studies, despite including a smaller sample size, showed no flap losses in similar patient cohorts.[36,41,42]

Besides flap loss, contracture recurrence is one of the most important complications when treating

a burn contracture.[43] The available studies reporting this outcome showed either no or very rare occurrence of this complication.[40,42,44–46] Indeed, free flaps allow the transfer of abundant, healthy and well vascularized tissue, alleviating tension on the scar, supporting proper wound healing, and reducing the likelihood of scar contracture recurrence. However, it is paramount to remove all the contracted tissue, including the margins of the scar, and to release the underlying ligamentous and tendinous structures under the skin contractures. If not completely addressed, they might lead to a persistent contracture and functional limitation. Free flaps allow coverage of extensive resections and especially when large areas are involved in the contracture, they represent an optimal reconstructive option.[47]

PREFABRICATED FLAPS

In patients who have sustained extensive burns, there is frequently a limited availability of healthy skin available for complex reconstructive procedures in unique areas such as the head, neck, and hands. Reconstructing burn injuries on the face and neck represents one of the most challenging tasks in reconstructive surgery, due to both functional and aesthetic aspects.[48] Serious scarring and deformity can follow facial burns, especially when they are healed by secondary intention. Traditional strategies such as skin grafts often present issues including color mismatch and unpredictable deformities. Local flaps might be an option but in extensive burn, local flaps might be unavailable.

A useful strategy in these complex scenarios is prefabrication, which is a term that was first introduced in the 1970s.[49–51] This technique involves the engineering of an axial flap from local or distant tissue by introducing a vascular pedicle into a body of tissue followed by a transfer of this neovascularized tissue into the defect based on its recently

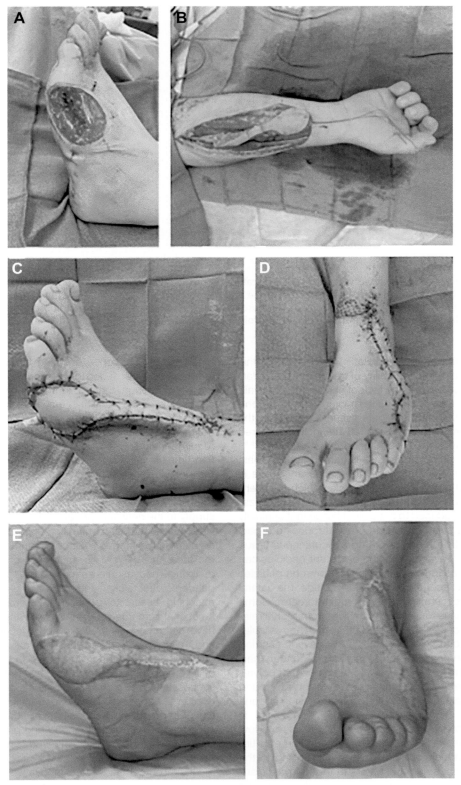

Fig. 1. 51-year-old male who sustained an electrical injury to the left foot. Following burn excision the defect involved exposure of the left fifth metatarsal bone and metatarsophalangeal joint (A). A right radial forearm free flap was harvested (B) and anastomosed to the left anterior tibial vessels (C, D). Three month follow up demonstrates a well healed flap with the full function of the foot (E, F).

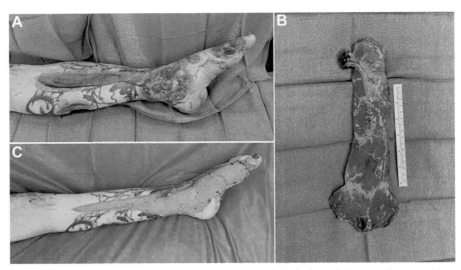

Fig. 2. 29-year-old male who sustained an electrical injury to the left foot. Following burn excision the defect involved exposure of the left first metatarsal bone and metatarsophalangeal joint, left tibia, ankle flexor and extensor tendons (*A*). A right rectus abdominis muscle free flap was harvested (*B*), anastomosed to the left posterior tibial vessels and skin grafted. One month follow up demonstrates a well healed flap and skin graft (*C*).

implanted vascular pedicle.[52] The benefit of this technique is first, the ability of transferring vascularized tissue despite the lack of flap donor site availability (due to extensive burn injuries), and second the ability to find the best tissue match, with the skin above the clavicle often being the preferred choice because of its unique characteristics.[48,53] The prefabrication process is carried out in 2 main stages. In the first stage, the necessary tissue is identified and a vascular pedicle, which is essentially a blood vessel that can foster neovascularization, is introduced to a recipient tissue that originally lacked a suitable pedicle, thus introducing a new axial pedicle to the overlying subcutaneous tissue and skin. A variety of local or distant pedicles can be used as for prefabrication.[52] Common pedicles used for free tissue transfer include the lateral femoral circumflex artery or radial forearm. Some studies have found that there is a proportional relationship of pedicle size and the rate of neovascularization and flap survival.[54] To prevent scarring around the pedicle and to facilitate secondary harvest of the prefabricated flap, a segment of polytetrafluoroethylene tubing can be wrapped around the pedicle. One may even consider using silicone or other nonadhesive sheeting.[52] The tissue is then kept in place for ideally 8 weeks to allow proper neovascularization.[52] The addition of a tissue expander facilitates easier flap raising in the subsequent stage and favors further neovascularization. The expander is generally filled until the desired volume is achieved. In the second stage, the fabricated flap is elevated, supported by new

blood supply networks, ensuring its viability and facilitating proper blood circulation in and out of the flap. Though there might be minor venous congestion issues initially, they typically resolve within the first 36 to 48 hours. In rare cases whereby congestion is severe, additional measures may be required including flap delay, lengthening maturation time, or increasing the contact area between the pedicle (usually in the form of a fascial flap) and the donor tissue.[52,55] By meticulously guiding the tissue development and ensuring a rich blood supply to the new flap, prefabrication seeks to provide a more natural, harmonized appearance in the reconstructive surgery of severe burn injuries on the face and neck. This method is grounded on fostering neovascularization, using tissue expanders effectively, and leveraging the best-matching tissue to optimize the aesthetic and functional outcomes of the surgery. Various studies have demonstrated its value and success. Pribaz and colleagues[48] shared their 10-year experience of prefabricated flaps in the head and neck. Out of 17 prefabricated flaps, 15 flaps were transferred successfully in 12 patients. Tissue expanders were used in 11 flaps and 7 flaps were transferred as free flaps. Zan and colleagues shared their 12-year experience using pre-expanded and prefabricated perforator flaps for total facial resurfacing in 42 patients demonstrating improved aesthetic and functional outcomes.[56] Other innovative prefabrication techniques have been further proposed including free prefabricated flaps with purely implanted arterialised venous loop,[57] prefabricated

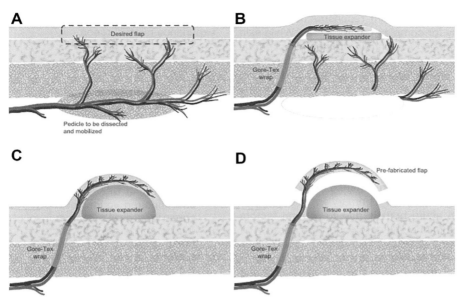

Fig. 3. Schematic diagram of the creation of prefabricated flaps. The desired flap is marked and the pedicle to be mobilized is identified (*A*); the pedicle is transposed to a recipient tissue that originally lacked a suitable pedicle, and it can be placed over a tissue expander (*B*); the expander is then filled until the desired volume is achieved (*C*); the fabricated flap is elevated and transferred to the desired location (*D*).

tissue-engineered Integra free flaps.[58] Many more applications have been used and often utilized in combination with prelamination, which demonstrates that this technique should remain the plastic surgeon's armamentarium when considering complex reconstructive challenges (**Fig. 3**).

PRELAMINATED FLAPS

The term prelaminatation was proposed by Pribaz and colleagues[59] referring to the implantation of tissue or other devices into a vascular territory prior to its transfer. The aim of prelamination is to modify a primary axial flap into a layered flap by incorporating the necessary support and lining components essential for composite reconstruction.

The first prelaminated flaps were forehead flaps prelaminated with bone and cartilage for nasal reconstruction. This technique was first attributed to Lexner in 1914, as mentioned by Denecke and Meyer, when he used tibial bone to prelaminate a forehead flap for reconstructing the nose.[59]

Prelamination is a two-stage procedure, in which a complex multilayered flap is created with the addition of grafts of different tissues and designed with a known vascular territory, and subsequently transferred through a microvascular anastomosis. This differs from prefabricated flaps because in a prelaminated flap the graft material is integrated into a pre-existing vascular territory, while prefabricated flaps are designed on a newly created vascular territory.

Prelamination of a flap at a distant site can provide the layers needed for the reconstruction of extensive and complex defects and they are used predominantly for facial defects.[53] Prelaminated flaps respond to the need of bringing tissue able to framework, lining and support at first stage. The tissue used include cartilage, bone, and porous polythene scaffolds, and bioabsorbable scaffolds. Refinements are often needed but can be accomplished secondarily. In addition, prelaminated flaps offer the advantage of simultaneously reconstruct adjacent structures. In particular, they offer unique advantages in case of complex defects whereby it is necessary to reconstruct also areas surrounding the nose, such as nasolabial folds, the lip or the cheek.[60] The forearm is the most commonly used site for flap prelamination but other flaps have also been used. Both radial and ulnar arterial territories can be used and the thin skin and the reliable vascular supply facilitate the incorporation of grafts. Despite the complexity and the number of surgeries often required, including revision and debulking procedures, prelaminated flaps represent a durable and satisfactory reconstructive option for complex defects, especially when involving multiple subunits of the face.

SUMMARY

In summary, microsurgery emerges as a crucial instrument for delivering exceptional care in both acute and delayed burn reconstructive surgery, particularly for complex patient cases. While skin grafting remains the primary treatment for partial and full-thickness burns, the need for more advanced strategies arises in severe burns associated with large and deep areas of soft tissue compromise and limb-threatening situations. In such cases, flap reconstruction, including microsurgical techniques, becomes essential for providing robust and reliable coverage, and minimizing complications. Today, flap reconstruction is rarely used in burn reconstruction, especially in the acute setting. The reluctance to use microsurgical reconstruction as a primary approach for patients with acute burn is due to several factors including the inherently prolonged the duration of free flap reconstruction, the need for a meticulous care and strict patient compliance in the postoperative period, the need of a specialized training, and the high risk of free flap failure in acute burns reported in literature. However, in some instances microsurgical reconstruction may remain the only reconstructive option, therefore further efforts are needed to improve surgical outcomes and obtain the best possible management of these rare but challenging patients. It is likely that the inflammatory sprout which follows the severe burn injury increases the risk for microvascular complications. Indeed, free flaps performed after 21 days from the day of injury (once the inflammatory cascade has settled down) demonstrated a higher probability of free flap survival. Further strategies to improve surgical outcomes involve preoperative optimization, including clinical and nutritional factors, nerve blocks, and careful management of organ support. Postoperatively, anticoagulation protocols are crucial, along with measures to optimize venous outflow and arterial inflow.

In delayed burn reconstruction, microsurgical reconstruction plays a key role in functional restoration, aesthetic improvement, and pain alleviation. Unlike in acute burns, the risk of flap loss in delayed reconstructive procedures is comparable to other elective patient populations. Microsurgical free flaps proved effective in minimizing the risk of contracture recurrence and maximizing the functional restoration, providing abundant, healthy, and well-vascularized tissue for optimal wound healing.

In complex facial reconstruction, the use of prefabricated and prelaminated flaps have expanded even more the tools available for reconstructive surgeons, demonstrating significant improvements in burn survivors quality of life in cases not curable with conventional free flaps. However, the technical difficulty of prefabricated and prelaminated flaps necessitates a meticulous

preoperative planning in addition to a skilled and experience microsurgeon.

CLINICS CARE POINTS

- In acute burn injuries, the risk of free flap failure is influenced by various factors, including local and systemic hyperinflammatory states. Burn-induced vascular changes, such as increased permeability and disrupted integrity, can lead to edema, compressive forces, and impaired venous outflow. Strategies to enhance surgical outcomes involve preoperative optimization, including clinical and nutritional support, nerve blocks, and organ support. Careful intraoperative and postoperative anticoagulation is crucial. Timing of reconstruction plays a significant role, with the highest flap failure risk between days 5 and 21 postinjury. Further research is needed to evaluate the influence of burn etiology and location on reconstructive outcomes and improve surgical strategies.

- Burn contracture free flap reconstruction demonstrates free flap failure rates similar to those observed in other elective patient populations. The use of free flaps reduces the risk of contracture recurrence by supplying ample, well-vascularized tissue that facilitates optimal wound healing and mitigates tension on the scar. It is imperative, however, to meticulously remove contracted fibrotic tissue and address underlying structures to prevent persistent contractures and associated functional limitations.

- Prefabrication emerges as a valuable strategy for facial reconstruction, involving the preparation of optimal tissue for transfer. This technique, carried out in 2 stages, introduces a vascular pedicle for neovascularization and uses tissue expanders to facilitate flap raising. Prefabrication aims for a more natural appearance and improved functional outcomes in severe burn reconstructive surgery. Studies have demonstrated its success, leveraging factors such as neovascularization, tissue expanders, and careful tissue development.

- Prelaminated flaps address the requirement for initial tissue providing framework, lining, and support. Secondary refinements are often necessary. Prelamination is primarily used for nose reconstruction but it allows the simultaneous reconstruction of adjacent structures, particularly beneficial in complex cases involving areas around the nose, such as naso-labial folds, the lip, or the cheek.

DISCLOSURE

The authors have no disclosures.

REFERENCES

1. Yakupu A, Zhang J, Dong W, et al. The epidemiological characteristic and trends of burns globally. BMC Publ Health 2022;22(1):1596.
2. Serror K, Boccara D, Chaouat M, et al. Dermal substitute: a safe and effective way in surgical management of adults post-burn dorsal foot contractures. Eur Rev Med Pharmacol Sci 2023;27(3 Suppl):29–36.
3. Hill DM, Hickerson WL, Carter JE. A risk-benefit review of Currently used dermal substitutes for burn wounds. J Burn Care Res 2023;44(Suppl_1):S26–32.
4. Jabir S, Frew Q, Magdum A, et al. Microvascular free tissue transfer in acute and secondary burn reconstruction. Injury 2015;46(9):1821–7.
5. Koul AR, Patil RK, Philip VK. Early use of microvascular free tissue transfer in the management of electrical injuries. Burns 2008;34(5):681–7.
6. Alessandri Bonetti M, Jeong T, Stofman GM, et al. A 10-year single-burn Center review of free tissue transfer for burn-related injuries. J Burn Care Res 2023. https://doi.org/10.1093/jbcr/irad132. irad132.
7. Bittner EA, Shank E, Woodson L, et al. Acute and perioperative care of the burn-injured patient. Anesthesiology 2015;122(2):448–64.
8. Baumeister S, Köller M, Dragu A, et al. Principles of microvascular reconstruction in burn and electrical burn injuries. Burns 2005;31(1):92–8.
9. Sauerbier M, Ofer N, Germann G, et al. Microvascular reconstruction in burn and electrical burn injuries of the severely traumatized upper extremity. Plast Reconstr Surg 2007;119(2):605–15.
10. Perrault D, Rochlin D, Pham C, et al. Timing of flap surgery in acute burn patients does not Affect complications. J Burn Care Res 2020;41(5):967–70.
11. Garner WL, Magee W. Acute burn injury. Clin Plast Surg 2005;32(2):187–93.
12. Levin LS. The reconstructive ladder. An orthoplastic approach. Orthop Clin North Am 1993;24(3):393–409.
13. Alessandri-Bonetti M, David J, Egro FM. Pedicled Latissimus Dorsi flap for extensive Scalp reconstruction in acute burns. Plast Reconstr Surg Glob Open 2023;11(8):e5217.
14. Shen TY, Sun YH, Cao DX, et al. The use of free flaps in burn patients: experiences with 70 flaps in 65 patients. Plast Reconstr Surg 1988;81(3):352–7.
15. Pan CH, Chuang SS, Yang JY. Thirty-eight free fasciocutaneous flap transfers in acute burned-hand injuries. Burns 2007;33(2):230–5.
16. Kasmirski JA, Alessandri-Bonetti M, Liu H, et al. Free flap failure and complications in acute burns: a systematic review and meta-analysis. Plast Reconstr Surg Glob Open 2023;11(10):e5311.
17. Yang Q, Ren ZH, Chickooree D, et al. The effect of early detection of anterolateral thigh free flap crisis on the salvage success rate, based on 10 years of experience and 1072 flaps. Int J Oral Maxillofac Surg 2014;43(9):1059–63.
18. Mücke T, Ritschl LM, Roth M, et al. Predictors of free flap loss in the head and neck region: a four-year retrospective study with 451 microvascular transplants at a single centre. J Cranio-Maxillo-Fac Surg 2016;44(9):1292–8.
19. Asif B, Rahim A, Fenner J, et al. Blood vessel occlusion in peri-burn tissue is secondary to erythrocyte aggregation and mitigated by a fibronectin-derived peptide that limits burn injury progression. Wound Repair Regen 2016;24(3):501–13.
20. DeSpain K, Rosenfeld CR, Huebinger R, et al. Carotid smooth muscle contractility changes after severe burn. Sci Rep 2021;11(1):18094.
21. Meizoso JP, Ray JJ, Allen CJ, et al. Hypercoagulability and venous thromboembolism in burn patients. Semin Thromb Hemost 2015;41(1):43–8.
22. Sherren PB, Hussey J, Martin R, et al. Acute burn induced coagulopathy. Burns 2013;39(6):1157–61.
23. Guilabert P, Martin N, Usúa G, et al. Coagulation alterations in Major burn patients: a Narrative review. J Burn Care Res 2023;44(2):280–92.
24. Pessoa Vaz M, Brandão C, Meireles R, et al. The role of microsurgical flaps in primary burn reconstruction. Ann Burns Fire Disasters 2018;31(3):233–7.
25. Pedrazzi N, Klein H, Gentzsch T, et al. Predictors for limb amputation and reconstructive management in electrical injuries. Burns 2022. https://doi.org/10.1016/j.burns.2022.08.007. S0305-4179(22)00208-X.
26. Alessandri-Bonetti M, Kasmirski JA, Liu HY, et al. Impact of Microsurgical Reconstruction Timing on the Risk of Free Flap Loss in Acute Burns: A Systematic Review and Meta-Analysis. Plast Reconstr Surg Glob Open. in pres.
27. van Zuijlen P, Gardien K, Jaspers M, et al. Tissue engineering in burn scar reconstruction. Burns Trauma 2015;3:18.
28. Finnerty CC, Jeschke MG, Branski LK, et al. Hypertrophic scarring: the greatest unmet challenge after burn injury. Lancet 2016;388(10052):1427–36.
29. Parrett BM, Pomahac B, Orgill DP, et al. The role of free-tissue transfer for head and neck burn reconstruction. Plast Reconstr Surg 2007;120(7):1871–8.
30. Chiang RS, Borovikova AA, King K, et al. Current concepts related to hypertrophic scarring in burn injuries. Wound Repair Regen 2016;24(3):466–77.
31. Dodd H, Fletchall S, Starnes C, et al. Current concepts burn Rehabilitation, Part II: Long-term Recovery. Clin Plast Surg 2017;44(4):713–28.

32. Orgill DP, Ogawa R. Current methods of burn reconstruction. Plast Reconstr Surg 2013;131(5): 827e–36e.

33. Deitch EA, Wheelahan TM, Rose MP, et al. Hypertrophic burn scars: analysis of variables. J Trauma 1983;23(10):895–8.

34. Dunkin CSJ, Pleat JM, Gillespie PH, et al. Scarring occurs at a critical depth of skin injury: precise measurement in a graduated dermal scratch in human volunteers. Plast Reconstr Surg 2007;119(6): 1722–32.

35. Friedstat JS, Hultman CS. Hypertrophic burn scar management: what does the evidence show? A systematic review of randomized controlled trials. Ann Plast Surg 2014;72(6):S198–201.

36. Kalra GS, Kalra S, Gupta S. Resurfacing in facial burn Sequelae using Parascapular free flap: a Long-term experience. J Burn Care Res 2022; 43(4):808–13.

37. Lj L, Jy Y, Fc W. Free flap transfer in burn reconstruction. Changgeng yi xue za zhi 1991;14(1). Available at: https://pubmed.ncbi.nlm.nih.gov/ 2039975/. [Accessed 10 December 2023].

38. Angrigiani C, Artero G, Sereday C, et al. Refining the extended circumflex scapular flap for neck burn reconstruction: a 30-year experience. J Plast Reconstr Aesthet Surg 2017;70(9):1252–60.

39. De Lorenzi F, van der Hulst R, Boeckx W. Free flaps in burn reconstruction. Burns 2001;27(6):603–12.

40. Ohkubo E, Kobayashi S, Sekiguchi J, et al. Restoration of the anterior neck surface in the burned patient by free groin flap. Plast Reconstr Surg 1991; 87(2):276–84.

41. Chang LS, Kim YH, Kim SW. Reconstruction of burn scar contracture deformity of the extremities using thin thoracodorsal artery perforator free flaps. ANZ J Surg 2021;91(9):E578–83.

42. Bali ZU, Özkan B, Keçeci Y, et al. Reconstruction of burn contractures with free anterolateral thigh flap in various anatomic sites. Ulus Travma Acil Cerrahi Derg 2021;27(3):337–43.

43. Liu HY, Alessandri Bonetti M, Kasmirski JA, et al. Free flap failure and contracture recurrence in delayed burn reconstruction: a systematic review and meta-analysis. Plast Reconstr Surg Glob Open, in pres.

44. Tsai FC, Mardini S, Chen DJ, et al. The classification and treatment algorithm for post-burn cervical contractures reconstructed with free flaps. Burns 2006; 32(5):626–33.

45. Woo SH, Seul JH. Optimizing the correction of severe postburn hand deformities by using aggressive

46. Angrigiani C. Aesthetic microsurgical reconstruction of anterior neck burn deformities. Plast Reconstr Surg 1994;93(3):507–18.

47. Seth AK, Friedstat JS, Orgill DP, et al. Microsurgical burn reconstruction. Clin Plast Surg 2017;44(4): 823–32.

48. Pribaz JJ, Fine N, Orgill DP. Flap prefabrication in the head and neck: a 10-year experience. Plast Reconstr Surg 1999;103(3):808–20.

49. Erol OO. The transformation of a free skin graft into a vascularized pedicled flap. Plast Reconstr Surg 1976;58(4):470–7.

50. Yao ST. Vascular implantation into skin flap: experimental study and clinical application: a preliminary report. Plast Reconstr Surg 1981;68(3):404–10.

51. Yao ST. Microvascular transplantation of prefabricated free thigh flap. Plast Reconstr Surg 1982; 69(3):568.

52. Guo L, Pribaz JJ. Clinical flap prefabrication. Plast Reconstr Surg 2009;124(6 Suppl):e340–50.

53. Pribaz JJ, Weiss DD, Mulliken JB, et al. Prelaminated free flap reconstruction of complex central facial defects. Plast Reconstr Surg 1999;104(2): 357–65 [discussion: 366–7].

54. Tark KC, Shaw WW. The revascularization interface in flap prefabrication: a quantitative and morphologic study of the relationship between carrier size and surviving area. J Reconstr Microsurg 1996; 12(5):325–30.

55. Daugherty THF, Pribaz JJ, Neumeister MW. The Use of prefabricated flaps in burn reconstruction. Clin Plast Surg 2017;44(4):813–21.

56. Zan T, Gao Y, Li H, et al. Pre-expanded, prefabricated Monoblock perforator flap for total facial resurfacing. Clin Plast Surg 2017;44(1):163–70.

57. Hoang NT, Staudenmaier R, Hai LH, et al. Successful re-construction of a large tissue defect using a free pre-fabricated flap with purely implanted arterialised venous loop. J Plast Reconstr Aesthet Surg 2009;62(7):e225–8.

58. Houle JM, Neumeister MW. A prefabricated, tissue-engineered Integra free flap. Plast Reconstr Surg 2007;120(5):1322–5.

59. Pribaz JJ, Fine NA. Prelamination: defining the prefabricated flap–a case report and review. Microsurgery 1994;15(9):618–23.

60. Mathy JA, Pribaz JJ. Prefabrication and prelamination applications in current aesthetic facial reconstruction. Clin Plast Surg 2009;36(3):493–505.

Management of the Sequelae of Skin Grafting
Pruritis, Folliculitis, Pigmentation Changes, and More

Anna White, MD[a], Debra Ann Reilly, MD[b],*

KEYWORDS

- Burn • Scar • Pruritis • Folliculitis • Hypertrophic scar • Hypopigmentation • Hyperpigmentation

KEY POINTS

- Pruritus, folliculitis, and pigment changes are common long-term sequelae of burns.
- Pruritus can range in severity, has lasting physical and psychological impacts on patients, and has multiple proposed mechanisms.
- Folliculitis is a concerning driver of infection in burn patients and has prophylactic, temporary, and permanent solutions that can be recommended.
- Pigment changes can vary based on the patient but overall prevalence is high, and there is a need for further investigation into effective treatment options.

PRURITUS
Introduction

Pruritus, also known as itch, is a common sequela of burns that can cause discomfort and distress and may last years following an initial burn injury. Although the causes of postburn pruritus (PBP) are still being investigated, the consequences are becoming increasingly well known and affecting millions of burn survivors each year. The incidence of annual burns that are severe enough to require medical care in the general global population is between 7 and 12 million people.[1] PBP most frequently begins early during the healing process, and epidemiologic evidence has recently revealed up to 93% of burn survivors experience daily itching 6 months after discharge. Unfortunately, PBP does not always resolve even long after the damaged tissue has been reepithelialized. This leads to 67% of patients reporting continued itching even 2 years after their burn injury.[2] Some studies have even found a prevalence rate of 40% 12 years after initial injury.[3]

Although itching may seem like a trivial symptom, the itching associated with PBP has the potential to significantly affect patients' lives. This includes disturbances in patient's sleep, self-inflicted injuries from scratching, and negative psychosocial effects. One population-based cohort study followed burn patients for 14 years after their injuries and found the incidence rate of sleep disorders in burn patients to be significantly higher than that of the general population, naming pruritis as one of the main inciting factors.[4] The risk of a secondary or ongoing injury is also a concern with severe itching. Scratching newly grafted skin can impede healing and add increased risk of infection.[5] However, patients whose grafts are healed or scars have matured are still at risk because they have been documented to experience itch causing them to scratch to the point of bleeding.[6] Finally, the psychosocial factors stem from severe itch impacting activities of daily living. This can lead to negative impacts on the mental health of burn survivors contributing to both posttraumatic stress disorder and depression.[5,7] The

[a] Department of Surgery, University of Nebraska Medical Center, Omaha, NE 68198-3280, USA; [b] Department of Surgery (Plastic), University of Nebraska Medical Center, 1430 South 85th Avenue, Omaha, NE 68124, USA
* Corresponding author.
E-mail address: dareilly@unmc.edu

Clin Plastic Surg 51 (2024) 409–418
https://doi.org/10.1016/j.cps.2023.12.004

large incidence and prevalence of PBP, coupled with the life changing effects it has on patients' lives, underscores the significance of addressing PBP as an integral part of comprehensive burn care.

Cause

Pruritis, in general, can have several causes, and there is an ongoing discussion on the classification of PBP. Recent studies have proposed categorizing PBP based on various pathophysiologic mechanisms including cutaneous, neuropathic, neurogenic, mixed, or psychogenic pruritus.[8] Those mechanisms and corresponding hypothesis for their role in PBP will be discussed in a later section.

Although the exact cause is not well understood, significant prognostic factors can highlight which patients are more at risk for developing PBP. Primarily, deeper thickness of burn has been correlated with increased likelihood of severe itch. Additionally, burns affecting the deep dermal layer and burns with increased total body surface area (TBSA) burned were more likely to result in PBP. %TBSA grafted also had a positive correlation with an increased rate of developing PBP symptoms. Female gender, presence of early acute traumatic stress symptoms, increased the number of surgeries needed, and burns to the limbs or face were also significant risk factors.[2,3]

Pathophysiology

To better understand how PBP originates, it is important to outline the mechanisms that induce pruritus in these patients in the first place. A review of the literature done in 2018 by Nedelec and colleagues proposed that PBP is primarily a combination of cutaneous and neuropathic itch.[9]

Cutaneous pruritus is seen in diseases such as dermatitis and is characterized by itching that originates from an external stimulus. It is sensed via nociceptive C-fibers in the skin. Unlike the C-fibers that detect pain, which are anatomically identical, those that detect pruritus are sensitive to different stimuli such as itch-inducing substances, such as histamine. Those C-fibers then send a signal through the spinothalamic tract to the ventromedial and dorsomedial thalamus, which leads to the urge to scratch.[3] Burn survivors have been found to have elevated histamine levels in their plasma as well as increased mast cells seen on histopathology.[9,10] Histopathologic examination of burn scar also demonstrates thicker epidermis, increased collagen bundles, and less elastic fibers.[3,9,10] Elevated mast cells and histamine strongly support a cutaneous element to PBP;

however, burn survivors do not respond as well to antihistamine medications as patients who suffer from other conditions that induce cutaneous pruritus. This points to a possible secondary or multifactorial cause of itch.

Neuropathic pruritus in burn patients is poorly understood; however, it is postulated that the initial burn injury could sensitize the nociceptors. This hypothesis of peripheral sensitization is based on our understanding of neuropathic pain because the pathophysiology of neuropathic itch is not well studied.[3] The strongest support for a neuropathic component to PBP is seen in patient's responsiveness to medications that treat classic neuropathic pain such as gabapentin, pregabalin, or naltrexone. Additionally, PBP is often accompanied by symptoms more often seen in neuropathic pain such as the description of "pins and needles."[9] These unique and sometimes complex constellations of symptoms, which vary patient to patient, support the hypothesis that multiple causes contribute to PBP. It also further highlights the need for individualized treatment of PBP (**Figs. 1** and **2**).

Presentation

Acute PBP begins at closure of the wound and continues through the first 6 months.[11] This is the time period where the largest percentage of patients will present as they begin to experience itching (up to 87% on average). Additionally, the acute phase is more likely to include severe symptoms.[3] The most intense pruritus is experienced during the proliferative phase of wound healing.[12] Chronic PBP is defined as itching experienced by burn patients 6 months after the burn has healed.[11]

Qualitative and quantitative assessment of pruritus with the use of standardized instruments is crucial in clinical practice for planning therapeutic interventions and accurately characterizing response to treatment. However, postburn pruritis is difficult to assess due to variation of the experience in adult and pediatric burn patients. Although there is currently no agreed upon tool for measuring the severity of pruritis in burn patients, the literature describes a variety of instruments to assess pruritus with some of the most used being the visual analog scale (VAS), numerical rating scale (NRS), and the verbal rating scale (VRS). These scales measure the subjective intensity of pruritus at a given time. The itch man scale (IMS) is another instrument that provides an NRS ranging from 0 to 4 combined with a pictorial element to denote interference with daily activities.

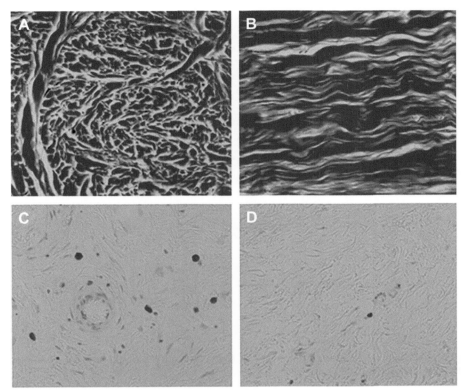

Fig. 1. (*left*). There are increased thin collagen bundles in the dermis of patients with PBP (*A*) compared with the thick collagen bundles in patients without PBP (*B*). There is also mast cell infiltration seen in the dermis of patients with PBP (*C*) compared with those without (*D*). (*From* Kwak IS, Park SY, Choi YH, et al. Clinical and Histopathological Features of Post Burn Pruritus: J Burn Care Res. 2016;37(6):343-349.)

It is important to explore a broad differential diagnosis when a patient presents with PBP. The first step should include a thorough physical examination to establish a well-defined location of the itching. Next, determine whether it is localized to the burn scar or if it is present more diffusely. Workup should also include a review of the patients' medications. Burn patients take a combination of several drugs including antibiotics that can cause allergic reactions, which can also manifest as pruritus. Additionally, an in-depth history can reveal any underlying dermatologic disorders such as atopic dermatitis or psoriasis that can manifest with similar pruritus (**Figs. 3–5**).

Treatments

An array of treatments exists to alleviate pruritus in patients suffering from burns; however, there is no consensus yet to which is most effective. The complex causes of PBP, which evolve over time, require individualized treatment regimens that are adjusted as patients heal. Although there is no consensus for the optimal treatment, there is fortunately a plethora of publications reviewing treatment protocols and offering physicians a rich resource of options. These treatments can be classified as either temporary or permanent and encompass oral medications, topical therapies, and physical modalities.

The current mainstay of treatment of PBP is topical emollients and both oral as well as antihistamines, which are massaged into the skin. Emollients and moisturizers are helpful given that deep partial-thickness burns or full-thickness burns will damage the sebaceous glands leading to dry skin.[9] Some studies found compression garments and pressure dressings to be helpful but only in the first year following injury. Massage alone was found to be a dissatisfying treatment compared with placebo for any patient with more than mild itching according to a randomized, blinded trial.[9] As for antihistamines, there is a wide range of response levels. According to one study, 20% of patients experienced complete relief; however, another 20% experienced no relief.[13,14] One double-blind, randomized, crossover trial compared antihistamines giving patients either diphenhydramine or ondansetron. The ondansetron was more effective, and an extended course proved to be more helpful than a one-time dose.[15]

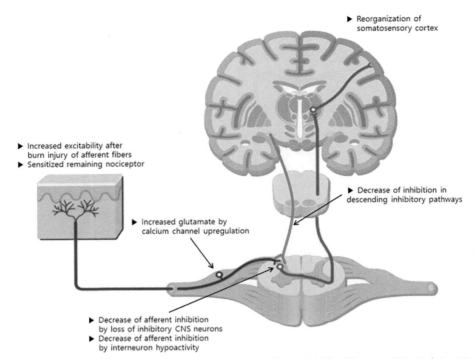

▶ Reorganization of
somatosensory cortex

▶ Increased excitability after
burn injury of afferent fibers
▶ Sensitized remaining nociceptor

▶ Decrease of inhibition in
descending inhibitory pathways

▶ Increased glutamate by
calcium channel upregulation

▶ Decrease of afferent inhibition
by loss of inhibitory CNS neurons
▶ Decrease of afferent inhibition
by interneuron hypoactivity

Fig. 2. (*right*). Proposed neuropathic pathway for PBP. (*From* Chung BY, Kim HB, Jung MJ, et al. Post-Burn Pruritus. Int J Mol Sci. 2020;21(11):3880.)

More permanent treatments that are being investigated include laser treatments. A meta-analysis recently investigated the effect of fractional carbon dioxide laser in the treatment of burn scars. This measured several aspects of burn scars, which improved after treatment, including both pain and pruritus improving by 20%.[16]

CLINICS CARE POINTS

- Keep your differential broad. Do not forget to rule out drug allergies, alternative dermatologic conditions, and other sensory-neural disorders such as peripheral neuropathy.
- Use effective tools to quantify severity of itch including the IMS.
- PBP responds well to agents that treat nerve pain, that is, gabapentin.
- Ondansetron has been shown to be a more effective antihistamine than diphenhydramine.

FOLLICULITIS
Introduction

Folliculitis is a dermatologic condition that is defined as an infection of the hair follicle. The source of the infection is most commonly bacterial but can also occur with fungal, viral, or even parasitic infections.[17] Folliculitis is a common and painful sequela of burns; however, it is underreported in the literature, and therefore, we do not have protocolized treatment algorithms.

There is no known change in risk for postburn folliculitis based on demographic features such as gender, age, or race. All patients are at risk for folliculitis. The mechanism of the burn has also not been showed to change the risk for developing folliculitis.[18] There have however been shown to be an increased incidence in the beard area in men, denser hair-bearing areas such as the chest or scalp, African Americans, children, or patients with scalp donor sites.

Folliculitis can affect patients with superficial to deep burns in any hair-bearing areas. Patients with recent burns, or patients with previously healed sites, are both susceptible. One burn center followed burn patients from the time of admission until their discharge from the burn unit to investigate infection rates. They found 27% of patients were identified to experience folliculitis during their hospitalization.[19] Given that infection is the most common cause of morbidity and mortality among burn patients, there should be a focus on decreasing incidence of folliculitis in burn patients in an effort to decrease overall risk of infection and therefore improve outcomes for burn victims.[20]

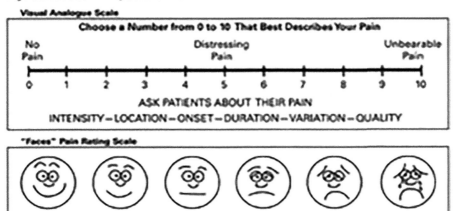

Fig. 3. VAS and NRS.

Cause

Burn injuries can damage hair follicles, creating small breaks in the skin where bacteria can multiply, leading to higher risk of the development of subsequent folliculitis. Patients who suffer burns from any area with hair growth are at risk for developing folliculitis, which can often be painful. Patients are most at risk, according to one study, if they have burns affecting greater than 20% of their TBSA.[19] It is hypothesized that partial-thickness burns may increase the risk for patients because the epidermis and part of the dermis is destroyed but hair follicles and their respective bacteria are preserved.[19] Other risk factors include immunosuppression, which can lead to infections from opportunistic organisms.

Pathophysiology

Folliculitis, in general, begins with inflammation in the hair follicle leading to pustules on the skin in hair-bearing areas. It can be broken down into 2 large subcategories: infectious and noninfectious. Noninfectious causes can occur secondary to trauma to the follicle or a blockage of the follicle. However, infectious causes are more common. Infectious folliculitis can be further divided into 4 categories: bacterial, fungal, viral, and parasitic. In patients with folliculitis after burns, bacterial is the most common offending pathogen. However, if burn victims are immunosuppressed, this can put them at an increased risk for fungal or viral folliculitis.

Burn patients often have trauma to hair follicles, either because of the burn itself or because of the trauma of treatments such as harvesting of a skin graft. This trauma leads to small defects in the skin.[21] These areas of injury allow bacteria and other pathogens to access the tissues and lead to infection of the hair follicles.[18] Not only is this new nidus for infection of great concern for burn patients but hair follicles also play a significant role in wound healing. Reepithelialization is made possible by the epidermal cells that regenerate from stem cells found in

Choose below the level of pain you are experiencing

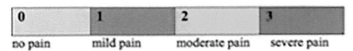

0. no pain or discomfort;

1. mild pain: feeling pain, but no oral medication (analgesic) is required;

2. moderate pain: feeling pain, but no oral medication (analgesic) is required;

3. Severe pain: feeling pain and is no longer able to perform any type of activity,

feeling the need to lie down and rest (analgesics have little or no effect on pain relief).

Fig. 4. VRS.

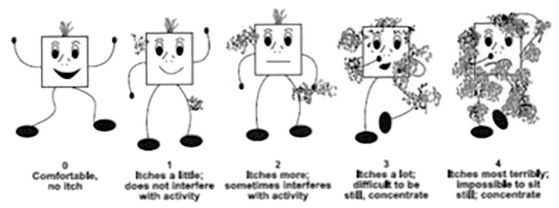

0	1	2	3	4
Comfortable, no itch	Itches a little; does not interfere with activity	Itches more; sometimes interferes with activity	Itches a lot; difficult to be still, concentrate	Itches most terribly; impossible to sit still; concentrate

Fig. 5. IMS, first developed by Blakeney and Marvin. This scale was developed for pediatric burn victims. (*From* Morris V, Murphy LM, Rosenberg M, Rosenberg L, Holzer CE, Meyer WJ. Itch Assessment Scale for the Pediatric Burn Survivor: J Burn Care Res. 2012;33(3):419-424.)

pilosebaceous follicles and migrate to the surface of a new wound.[22] Postburn folliculitis not only creates a new infection that must be treated in a patient but also inhibits wound healing. The most common pathogens responsible for folliculitis include coagulase-positive *Streptococcus*, *Staphylococcus aureus*, methicillin-resistant *Staphylococcus aureus*, and *Pseudomonas aeruginosa*.[18,21] Rarely, there are viral or fungal infections that can lead to folliculitis with pathogens such as *Candida* or *Malassezia*, and these are typically more common in immunosuppressed patients.

Presentation

Folliculitis will develop based on its area of presentation, and therefore, it can be subclassified as either folliculitis of the head and neck or folliculitis of the body. Folliculitis that develops on the body is more likely to present as red spots early on that develop into roughly 1-mm wide vesicles or pustules.[18,23] These pustules can then break open and develop crusts. They are most often small and superficial.[18] Folliculitis of the head

and scalp begins as small pustules, rather than red spots. These pustules form around individual hair follicles and then as they burst open, they also form a crust. Both forms of folliculitis can spread rapidly.

Folliculitis is primarily a diagnosis of exclusion, so adequate evaluation is important. Differential diagnosis may include diseases such as drug-induced folliculitis, acne vulgaris, or pseudo folliculitis barbae. Infectious folliculitis can spread quickly to other parts of the body, so a quick and thorough assessment is important. If suspicion for folliculitis is high, there should be cultures taken from the infected area of the wound in order to ensure appropriate treatment regimen[21] (**Fig. 6**).

Treatment

The management for folliculitis will greatly depend on cause. Typically, the inciting pathogen is bacterial, and antibiotic regimens can be tailored based on cultures. Unfortunately, there is not a standardized treatment algorithm for the management of

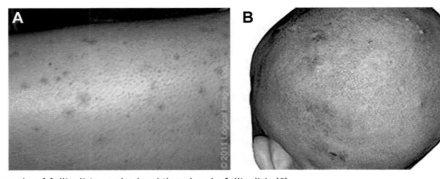

Fig. 6. Example of folliculitis on the leg (*A*) and scalp folliculitis (*B*).

postburn folliculitis specifically but there are broadly agreed on goals of treatment. These include removing the bacteria or offending pathogen from the wound and promoting healing to decrease the opportunity for future infection.

Treatment of folliculitis has traditionally involved gentle debridement of any crusting over the wounds followed by irrigation of the wound with a chlorhexidine or other aseptic solution. This treatment needs to be repeated frequently, and the regimen is cumbersome and painful for patients. After debridement and thorough cleaning, topical agents will be applied and are catered to the patient based on pathogen sensitivity. Examples of topical treatments include mupirocin ointment for gram-positive organisms such as *Staphylococcus* or *Streptococcus*, diluted acetic acid for *Pseudomonas*, or antifungals including azoles or permethrin. Some treatment protocols suggest soaking the area of folliculitis in vegetable oil before the treatment in order to more effectively remove the crusts that have formed.[21]

Patients with folliculitis that is refractory to other treatments may benefit from laser hair removal. Diode lasers that are used in burned areas can reduce hair density by more than half.[21] Diode lasers, among other laser hair removal devices, work by targeting melanin for selective photothermolysis, which destroys the hair follicle.[24] Several studies have evaluated the safety and efficacy of laser hair removal, deeming it both safe and the most effective method for permanent reduction in hair growth. One prospective study looking at long-term follow-up found that reduction rates ranged from 65% to 75% at the 20-month mark for patients.[25]

SUMMARY/CLINICS CARE POINTS

- All patients with burns in hair-bearing areas are at risk.
- Patients with partial-thickness burns may be at an increased risk.
- Folliculitis spreads to other areas of the body, and rapid diagnosis and treatment is important.
- Treatment should be tailored based on susceptibilities of infectious bacteria or pathogen.
- Preventative treatment with topical antibiotics is recommended in burn patients.

PIGMENT CHANGES
Introduction

Disorders of skin pigment change, whether it be hyperpigmentation or hypopigmentation, are the most common long-term sequelae of burns. According to the Journal of Burn Care, there is at least a temporary loss of pigment with all burns except first degree. These pigment changes can last months or can become permanent.[26] This leads to a large psychological impact on patients after surviving a burn injury.[27] The degree of pigmentation changes correlates with the depth of the burn and severity of skin damage. The scale of this problem is large, leading patients to low confidence and even isolation for some patients.[28] This problem, although widespread and distressing to many patients, is benign in nature; therefore, there is no gold standard treatment, and there has been a need in burn literature to further investigate pigment changes in burn patients.

Cause

To accurately describe the cause of pigment changes seen in burn patients, it is important to outline the location of melanin-producing cells, melanocytes, in the skin to correlate their response to varying degrees of burn injuries. Skin pigmentation is determined by 4 different pigments but melanin is the predominant one. It is found primarily at the lower aspect of the epidermis, in the stratum basale layer.[26] Therefore, any partial-thickness burn that damages the deeper layers of the epidermis will cause pigment changes but burn injuries are more likely to result in pigment changes in patients with Fitzpatrick type III-VI skin (**Fig. 7**).

Pathophysiology

The complete pathophysiology of postburn pigment changes has not been fully elucidated but it is thought to be linked to the role melanocytes play in wound healing. Melanocytes exist in the basal layer of the epidermis.[29,30] Normally, their role is to produce melanin, which is transported by melanosomes along their dendritic arms and delivered to keratinocytes. These melanocytes can be injured during partial-thickness or full-thickness burns. During a burn injury, the inflamed skin induces release of cytokines that have several effects, including proliferation of melanocytes and upregulation of melanogenesis. This may be responsible for some of the postburn hyperpigmentation.[31,32]

Hypopigmentation occurs more commonly in full-thickness burns. Because there is a loss

Type I	Type II	Type III	Type IV	Type V	Type VI
White skin. Always burns, never tans.	Fair skin. Always burns, tans with difficulty.	Average skin color. Sometimes mild burn, tan about average.	Light-brown skin. Rarely burns. Tans easily.	Brown skin. Never burns. Tans very easily.	Black skin. Heavily pigmented. Never burns, tans very easily.

Fig. 7. The Fitzpatrick skin classification. Patients with Fitzpatrick type III-VI are more likely to suffer from pigment changes after burn injury. (*From* Department of Surgical Oncology, Fox Chase Cancer Center, Philadelphia, PA, USA, Ward WH, Lambreton F, et al. Clinical Presentation and Staging of Melanoma. In: Department of Surgical Oncology, Fox Chase Cancer Center, Philadelphia,PA, USA, Ward WH, Farma JM, Department of Surgical Oncology, Fox Chase Cancer Center, Philadelphia,PA, USA, eds. Cutaneous Melanoma: Etiology and Therapy. Codon Publications; 2017:79-89.)

of melanocytes during a full-thickness injury, there are no melanocytes to deposit melanin into the healed burn wound. As the wound heals, scar tissue forms and may block any migration of melanocytes into the burned region.

One study looked at the presence of melanocytes after various wound depths in both partial-thickness and full-thickness wounds and found that melanocytes were completely repopulated in partial-thickness wounds at 35 days but not in full-thickness wounds.[33] The conclusion drawn from this study is that the deeper the wound, the slower the repigmentation. They also found melanocyte migration to the new epithelium will be delayed after reepithelialization by several weeks to months or even never.[26] The delay in the distribution of newly migrated melanocytes is not well known.

Presentation

As discussed in earlier sections, both partial-thickness and full-thickness burns are susceptible to pigment changes with healing. This most commonly presents as wounds that are pink from neovascularization or hypopigmented. It can then develop into hyperpigmentation after time or with sun exposure. This presentation can vary greatly depending on the patient's skin tone.

One group analyzed a sample of children who had sustained second-degree burns to examine their skin color. They found that during the first 3 years, burn site color changes among the patients were variable but after 3 years, there was a collective hyperpigmentation to the site of the healed burn.[34] They also found the degree of hyperpigmentation was positively correlated with preburn skin color (**Fig. 8**).

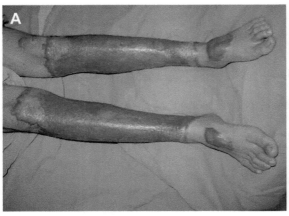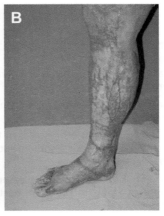

Fig. 8. Examples of hyperpigmentation (*A*) and hypopigmentation (*B*) after a burn. (*From* Dai NT, Chang HI, Wang YW, et al. Restoration of skin pigmentation after deep partial or full-thickness burn injury. Adv Drug Deliv Rev. 2018;123:155-164. https://doi.org/10.1016/j.addr.2017.10.010.)

Treatment and Prevention

The best treatment of pigment changes is preventative. Burn patients are cautioned to avoid sun exposure during the repigmentation period of wound healing because it can cause hyperpigmentation.[26] Sunscreen and protective clothing are recommended for all patients but especially those with healing burn scars. Although it is important for burn patients to try to go back to their normal lives, they can take precautions during peak sun hours to try and minimize the negative effects of ultraviolet radiation.

There are options for temporary as well as permanent treatments. Temporary treatments may include cover up, makeup, or tinted clothing. One literature review compared several treatment modalities and found topical agents seemed to be a common choice as first-line agent in hyperpigmentation. These agents included retinoids, triamcinolone, and salicylic acid. They found that overall topical tretinoin is an effective treatment of postburn hyperpigmentation. Methimazole was also studied as a depigmenting agent and was found to be effective.[35]

Permanent treatments include laser therapy for small areas as well as pulse dilators, which target hemoglobin in dilated capillaries. Laser treatment can disperse pigment in a hyperpigmented wound as well as stimulate melanocytes in a hypopigmented wound.[28] A more aggressive treatment option would be recreating the wound and placing a new skin graft to bring new pigment to the area.[26] For areas of hypopigmentation, permanent treatments include makeup or tattoos to camouflage.

CLINICS CARE POINTS

- Pigment changes will present differently based on the thickness of the burn as well as the skin tone of the patient.
- The best treatment is prevention of pigment changes as much as possible.
  o Avoid excess sun exposure.
  o Wear sun protective garments.
- Long-term treatments such as tattoos, laser therapy, or even a new skin graft have variable results and require more investigation.

DISCLOSURE

The authors have no disclosures to make.

REFERENCES

1. James SL, Lucchesi LR, Bisignano C, et al. Epidemiology of injuries from fire, heat and hot substances: global, regional and national morbidity and mortality estimates from the Global Burden of Disease 2017 study. Inj Prev 2020;26(Suppl 2):i36–45.
2. Carrougher GJ, Martinez EM, McMullen KS, et al. Pruritus in adult burn survivors: postburn prevalence and risk factors associated with increased intensity. J Burn Care Res 2013;34(1):94–101.
3. Chung BY, Kim HB, Jung MJ, et al. Post-burn pruritus. Int J Mol Sci 2020;21(11):3880.
4. Liang CY, Chen CC, Wang KY, et al. Increased risk for sleep disorders in burn patients: a 14-year nationwide, population-based cohort study. Burns 2021;47(6):1408–15.
5. Van Loey NEE, Bremer M, Faber AW, et al. The Research group. itching following burns: epidemiology and predictors. Br J Dermatol 2007;0(0). https://doi.org/10.1111/j.1365-2133.2007.08278.x. 071106220718003.
6. Gauffin E, Öster C, Gerdin B, et al. Prevalence and prediction of prolonged pruritus after severe burns. J Burn Care Res 2015;36(3):405–13.
7. McGarry S, Burrows S, Ashoorian T, et al. Mental health and itch in burns patients: potential associations. Burns 2016;42(4):763–8.
8. Twycross R, Greaves MW, Handwerker H, et al. Itch: scratching more than the surface. QJM 2003;96(1):7–26.
9. Nedelec B, LaSalle L. Postburn itch: a review of the literature. Wounds Compend Clin Res Pract 2018;30(1):E118–24.
10. Kwak IS, Park SY, Choi YH, et al. Clinical and histopathological features of post burn pruritus. J Burn Care Res 2016;37(6):343–9.
11. Parnell LKS, Nedelec B, Rachelska G, et al. Assessment of pruritus characteristics and impact on burn survivors. J Burn Care Res 2012;33(3):407–18.
12. Zachariah JR, Rao AL, Prabha R, et al. Post burn pruritus—a review of current treatment options. Burns 2012;38(5):621–9.
13. Morris V, Murphy LM, Rosenberg M, et al. Itch assessment scale for the pediatric burn survivor. J Burn Care Res 2012;33(3):419–24.
14. Vitale M, Fields-Blache C, Luterman A. Severe itching in the patient with burns. J Burn Care Rehabil 1991;12(4):330–3.
15. S Gross, Overbaugh, Jansen. Ondansetron for treating itch in healing burns. Internet J Pain Symptom Control Palliat Care. 5(1).
16. Zhang C, Yin K, Shen YM. Efficacy of fractional carbon dioxide laser therapy for burn scars: a meta-analysis. J Dermatol Treat 2021;32(7):845–50.
17. Winters RD, Mitchell M. Folliculitis. In: StatPearls. StatPearls. 2023. Available at: http://www.ncbi.nlm.nih.

gov/books/NBK547754/ 2023. Accessed September 18, 2023.

18. Folliculitis Following Burn Injury. https://www. hmpgloballearningnetwork.com/site/wounds/article/ 2657. Accessed September 18, 2023.

19. Ramirez-Blanco CE, Ramirez-Rivero CE, Diaz-Martinez LA, et al. Infection in burn patients in a referral center in Colombia. Burns 2017;43(3): 642–53.

20. Posluszny JA, Conrad P, Halerz M, et al. Surgical burn wound infections and their clinical implications. J Burn Care Res 2011;32(2):324–33.

21. Tay YT, Tang N, Department of Plastic Surgery, Eastern Health, Box Hill 3128, Australia, Department of Plastic Surgery, Eastern Health, Box Hill 3128, Australia, Ng SKH, Department of Plastic Surgery, Eastern Health, Box Hill 3128, Australia and Victoria Adult Burns Service, The Alfred, Melbourne 3004, Australia. Management of folliculitis in burn patients. Trichol Cosmetol Open J 2022;5(1):1–3.

22. Cotsarelis G. Epithelial stem cells: a folliculocentric view. J Invest Dermatol 2006;126(7):1459–68.

23. Luelmo-Aguilar J, bat Santandreu M. Folliculitis: recognition and management. Am J Clin Dermatol 2004;5(5):301–10.

24. Gupta G. Diode laser: permanent hair "reduction" not "removal". Int J Trichol 2014;6(1):34.

25. Lou WW, Quintana AT, Geronemus RG, et al. Prospective study of hair reduction by diode laser (800 nm) with long-term follow-up. Dermatol Surg 2000;26(5):428–32.

26. Greenhalgh DGA. Primer on pigmentation. J Burn Care Res 2015;36(2):247–57.

27. Lupon E, Laloze J, Chaput B, et al. Treatment of hyperpigmentation after burn: a literature review. Burns 2022;48(5):1055–68.

28. Chadwick S, Heath R, Shah M. Abnormal pigmentation within cutaneous scars: a complication of wound healing. Indian J Plast Surg 2012;45(02): 403–11.

29. Ward WH, Lambreton F, Farma JM, et al. Clinical presentation and staging of melanoma. In: Department of Surgical Oncology, Fox Chase Cancer Center, editors. Cutaneous melanoma: etiology and therapy. Philadelphia: Codon Publications; 2017. p. 79–89. https://doi.org/10.15586/codon.cutaneousmelanoma. 2017.ch6.

30. Paus R. Migrating melanocyte stem cells: masters of disaster? Nat Med 2013;19(7):818–9.

31. Taylor S, Grimes P, Lim J, et al. Postinflammatory hyperpigmentation. J Cutan Med Surg 2009;13(4): 183–91.

32. Dai NT, Chang HI, Wang YW, et al. Restoration of skin pigmentation after deep partial or full-thickness burn injury. Adv Drug Deliv Rev 2018; 123:155–64.

33. Chadwick SL, Yip C, Ferguson MWJ, et al. Repigmentation of cutaneous scars depends on original wound type. J Anat 2013;223(1):74–82.

34. De Chalain TMB, Tang C, Thomson HG. Burn area color changes after superficial burns in childhood: can they be predicted? J Burn Care Rehabil 1998; 19(1):39–49.

35. Kasraee B, Handjani F, Parhizgar A, et al. Topical methimazole as a new treatment for postinflammatory hyperpigmentation: report of the first case. Dermatology 2005;211(4):360–2.

Surgical Management of Chronic Neuropathic Burn Pain

Check for updates

Ying C. Ku, DO[a], Arya Andre Akhavan, MD[b],
Charles Scott Hultman, MD, MBA[c],*

KEYWORDS

• Burn • Neuropathic • Pain • Laser • Lipofilling • Nerve surgery • Surgical intervention

KEY POINTS

- Burn-related chronic neuropathic pain is defined as neuropathic pain persisting for at least 6 months following a burn injury and the diagnosis should be confirmed by 2 physicians.
- If initial medical management is ineffective, surgical intervention (laser, fat grafting, nerve decompression, neuroma excision, nerve transfer) is considered in patients with an anatomic cause of the pain.
- Nerve decompression should be contemplated in all patients presenting with motor involvement.
- Tinel's signs guide first-step surgical treatment: laser / fat grafting (0 or multiple Tinel's), nerve decompression (1–2 Tinel's proximal to or at the burn scar), and neuroma excision (1–2 Tinel's at the burn scar).
- Nerve transfer (targeted muscle reinnervation, regenerative peripheral nerve interfaces, and vascularized denervated muscle targets) is typically considered the last resort for patients who have failed other surgical interventions.

CHRONIC NEUROPATHIC PAIN

Chronic neuropathic pain (CNP) following burns, or burn-related nerve pain, arises either from the burn injury itself or, as a consequence of the management of the burn injury which leads to secondary nerve injury and irritation.[1–3] Signs and symptoms of CNP vary among patients and may include spontaneous or evoked pain, continuous or intermittent pain, and other manifestations including dysesthesia, paresthesia, weakness, numbness, Tinel's sign, altered temperature sensation, and pruritus.[2,4–6] The primary cause of neuropathic pain is attributed to lesions or pathologic conditions that disrupt the normal functionality of the somatosensory system.[5] In burn patients, this disruption occurs primarily in the form of nerve injury at the level of the peripheral nervous system. Such injury can be partial or complete, ranging from mononeuropathy to mononeuropathy multiplex and polyneuropathy.[7,8] Mononeuropathy results from injury to a single peripheral nerve, stemming from localized factors such as burns (heat, chemical, and electrical), iatrogenic causes (debridement, escharotomies/fasciotomies), compression (edema, delayed escharotomies, tight dressing, heterotopic ossification, incorrect splinting, hypertrophic scar, and nerve sheath hematoma), or dynamic, forceful physical therapy.[7,9–12] Mononeuropathy multiplex involves the

[a] Department of Surgery, Campbell University School of Osteopathic Medicine, 4350 US Highway 421 South, Lillington, NC 27546, USA; [b] Division of Plastic and Reconstructive Surgery, Department of Surgery, Rutgers New Jersey Medical School, 90 Bergen St., Newark, NJ 07103; [c] Department of Plastic and Reconstructive Surgery, WPP Plastic and Reconstructive Surgery, WakeMed Health and Hospitals, 3000 New Bern Avenue, Raleigh, NC 27610, USA
* Corresponding author. Department of Plastic and Reconstructive Surgery, WPP Plastic and Reconstructive Surgery, WakeMed Health and Hospitals, 3000 New Bern Avenue, Raleigh, NC 27610.
E-mail address: CHULTMAN@wakemed.org

Clin Plastic Surg 51 (2024) 419–434
https://doi.org/10.1016/j.cps.2024.02.009
0094-1298/24/© 2024 Elsevier Inc. All rights reserved.

dysfunction of 2 or more peripheral nerves in different areas of the body and is associated with more severe burns (>20% TBSA, > 15% full-thickness).[13,14] It is most commonly caused by a combination of localized and generalized factors, including metabolic conditions, drugs, sepsis, neurotoxins, multi-organ failure, and prolonged mechanical ventilation.[7,8,15-18] Lastly, polyneuropathy refers to abnormalities in numerous nerves in a distal symmetric pattern, resulting from a combination of generalized factors.[7,8,15-18] Notably, the presence of burn scars itself also presents a challenge, as dysregulated tissue repair and regeneration can further exacerbate underlying nerve injuries, contributing to the complexity of burn-related CNP.[19,20]

The prevalence of postburn CNP ranges from 6% to 82% among burn survivors.[2,8,14,21-27] This wide range may be attributed to differences in diagnostic methodologies, time of diagnosis, the course of injury, and recovery. Nevertheless, CNP is known to be associated with psychiatric morbidities and significantly impacts the quality of life (QoL) and long-term functional recovery.[22,25,28,29] However, given the diverse etiologies and clinical manifestation of the pain, there is no standardized approach for CNP. Furthermore, despite the availability of pharmacologic and medical therapies, these methods remain only partially effective for many patients. To date, there are limited studies in the literature investigating options for surgical intervention in patients with burn-related CNP.

RISK FACTORS AND PREDICTIVE MODEL

Several risk factors and predictors for burn-related CNP have been proposed in the literature, including older age, male sex, moderate-to-severe pain, substance/alcohol/tobacco use, greater full-thickness burns, greater %TBSA burns, presence of an upper arm or thigh burn, mechanical ventilation, surgical burn treatment, a greater number of surgical burn treatment, and a longer hospital length of stay (LOS).[1,2,25] Similar to the wide range in CNP prevalence, variations in risk factors/predictors may stem from differences in follow-up periods, assessment methods, and statistical analyses used in different studies. Interestingly, there is a difference in CNP predictors based on different anatomic locations of burns, with tobacco and substance use being relevant across most anatomic locations of the body.[1] Additionally, several factors were found to be associated with patients who progressed from having acute neuropathic pain to CNP, and these included greater % TBSA burns, greater full-thickness burns, a greater number of surgical burn treatment, and a higher number of complications.[30] A validated predictive model was developed to predict a patient's risk of developing CNP at 6 months postburn injury, and it consisted of age, tobacco use, substance abuse, alcohol abuse, upper arm burn, thigh burn, number of burn operations, and hospital LoS.[1] Identifying risk factors and using a predictive model can help proactively monitor patients at risk, provide education in advance, and establish appropriate expectations.

ASSESSMENT AND DIAGNOSIS

CNP is diagnosed clinically through subjective symptom reports and a physical examination assessing sensory (light touch, vibration, proprioception, two-point discrimination, and cold/heat tolerance) and motor functions (muscle strength).[4,24,31] Additionally, the Tinel test can help locate an irritated nerve, with positive signs indicating possible neuromas.[32] In general, burn-related CNP is defined as paresthesias and/or dysesthesias greater than 6 months following the initial burn injury, with clinical signs and symptoms independent of other illnesses or medications.[2] Two clinicians should confirm the diagnosis, and a trial of neuro-modulating medication should be attempted. Notably, it is crucial to differentiate CNP from other forms of chronic pain for proper management. Common patient complaints include electric shocks, hypersensitivity, allodynia, paresthesias, and numbness in the region of a known nerve distribution.[31] A detailed clinical examination is paramount to pinpoint the nerves causing pain. If the patient's pain does not align with a known nerve course, the likelihood of CNP is low. Diagnostic nerve blocks are a helpful modality to confirm and map out the location of injured nerve distribution, and symptom relief after blocks suggests nerve compression or the presence of neuroma.[31,33] Although electrodiagnostic studies (electromyography and nerve conduction velocity) have been used to monitor CNP,[34] their role in diagnosis is limited. Electrodiagnostic studies are relatively expensive, it can take a few weeks to set up the procedure, and some patients do not tolerate the lengthy procedure. Most importantly, scar areas are frequently not tested. These tests were not found to accurately predict CNP, especially in small fiber neuropathies.[4,15] Nevertheless, electrodiagnostic testing may provide utility in cases whereby the patient's presentation and physical examination do not consolidate a diagnosis, or if multiple nerves are suspected to be involved.[15] Lastly, MRI and high-resolution ultrasound (US) can identify and locate neuromas, nerve lesions, and nerve entrapment,[35-37] although their role in diagnosing burn-related CNP remains uncertain. Once CNP is diagnosed, pain level should be assessed and monitored using an objective pain assessment tool. Commonly used tools include the Visual Analogue Scale (VAS), the Numerical Rating Scale (NRS), the Verbal Rating Scale (VRS), and the Faces Pain Scale-Revised.[38] The NRS is often preferred due to its ease of use and higher compliance rates, with pain categorized as mild (1–3), moderate (4–6), and severe (7–10).[38] Regular assessments are crucial to evaluate responses to management, along with the characteristics and severity of CNP.

Finally, to better understand the pathology and identify optimal treatment options for the heterogeneous group of patients with burn-related CNP, a classification system consisting of 4 distinct groups, based on etiologies, was proposed.[3] These include direct nerve injury, nerve compression, electrical injury, and nerve dysfunction secondary to systemic injury. This system was developed considering burn injury characteristics, signs and symptoms, and the management of the burn injury. Using this classification system can help guide patient management and has been applied in research methods with the goal of improving pain outcomes in this patient population.

INITIAL MANAGEMENT - PHARMACOLOGIC AGENTS

Typically, a referral to pain management is recommended for all patients with CNP. A personalized pharmacologic regimen should be developed for each patient with a stepwise strategy, consisting of base management (gabapentin/pregabalin, duloxetine/amitriptyline, local/topical lidocaine, and vitamin C.) and adjuncts (regional or local blocks with lidocaine/bupivacaine, ketamine, and hydroxyzine).[39–42] Gabapentin and pregabalin inhibit calcium influx at nerve terminals, reducing the release of excitatory neurotransmitters. Duloxetine and amitriptyline increase circulating serotonin and norepinephrine levels, modulating endogenous analgesic mechanisms in the brain and spinal cord, contributing to the inhibition of pain signals. Lidocaine and bupivacaine act as sodium channel blockers, inhibiting depolarization and subsequent signal propagation. Vitamin C, an essential cofactor, plays a key role in the amidation of various peptides and is involved in numerous vital biological functions.[43] It has demonstrated effectiveness in reducing pain,[6] likely attributable to its antioxidant and anti-inflammatory properties.[43] Ketamine produces analgesia by modifying central nervous system pain signal processing, which includes inhibiting N-methyl-D-aspartate receptors and engaging other mechanisms such as descending

inhibition and exerting anti-inflammatory effects.[44] Hydroxyzine, an H1 receptor blocker, offers skeletal muscle relaxation, bronchodilation, antihistamine, antiemetic, and analgesic properties. It has demonstrated efficacy in reducing postoperative pain[45] and should be considered for CNP-associated pruritus.

In general, medications are initiated at lower doses and titrated gradually through a targeted multimodal approach.[39] Allow sufficient time for the medication to demonstrate optimal effects before considering discontinuation, as some may require weeks to months for assessment. Additionally, consider dose adjustments in alignment with the patient's renal and hepatic functions. Notably, opioids are not the first-line option for managing CNP due to limited benefits and a serious risk profile. As a general rule, a minimum effective dose for the shortest possible interval is preferred.[39] If discontinuation is necessary, medications should be tapered, if possible, to avoid abrupt discontinuation. Patients should be educated on the importance of adhering to the management plan, including following scheduled doses even in the absence of pain. Additionally, they should be informed about the risks of developing secondary chronic pain from prolonged use of medications.

INITIAL MANAGEMENT - NONPHARMACOLOGIC

While pharmacologic agents are essential in pain management, it is crucial to integrate nonpharmacologic medical management early on. This multimodal approach is essential for benefiting patients by addressing various psychophysiological pain pathways. A detailed discussion regarding different therapies is above the scope of this study, later in discussion we provided a brief overview of common management options.

Occupational Therapy and Physical Therapy

Physical and occupational therapies are integral to the functional recovery of burn patients, especially in the alleviation of chronic pain. Physical therapy (PT) involves exercises designed for gradual strength building and range of motion improvement, enhancing flexibility, mobility, and pain reduction.[46] Strength training is particularly important since muscle weakness resulting from nerve injury is frequently observed. Support devices such as splints or braces may be used to provide temporary immobility, thereby reducing movement in the affected area. Occupational therapy (OT) provides education and assistance for lifestyle modifications aimed at preventing and/or reducing pain, and ultimating improving day-to-day function.[47] They assume an essential role in a patient's daily functioning and offer consultations for coping strategies to the overall rehabilitation process.

Cutaneous Care

Optimizing scar management remains a priority in the treatment of burn pain, as neuropathic pain can arise from scar compression on peripheral nerves. Various strategies have been established for treating and preventing scars, encompassing the use of silicon gels, topical steroids (in gel, cream, or tape form), moisturizing agents, compression, sun protection, and scar massage.[48] Silicone sheets have been a longstanding and effective approach, reducing the itching and dryness of the scars while improving hydration. This method has demonstrated efficacy in both treating and preventing hypertrophic scars.[49] Similarly, transdermal steroid application (gel, cream, or tape) has demonstrated effectiveness in alleviating pain, reducing itchiness, and improving the overall appearance of pathologic scars.[50] Compression therapy is a well-established approach in scar management, with pressure believed to induce modifications in collagen fibers through various cellular processes.[51] This modality has been long used in burn care to prevent and/or treat pathologic scar formations. Lastly, sun protection and scar massage are imperative for optimal healing, with UV light avoidance recommended for at least a year to prevent damage and depigmentation to healing skin. Regular scar massage has been found to be effective in desensitizing scars and can be combined with stretching exercises to promote increased scar flexibility and softness.

Lymphatic Massage

Lymphatic circulation may become obstructed either directly due to the burn injury or as a consequence of subsequent scar compression. This obstruction can result in a cascade of dysfunctional microcirculation, including the irritation and inflammation of nerve endings.[52] To address this, lymphatic drainage massage can be performed to manually assist lymph flow, preventing fluid accumulation. In turn, this promotes the normal circulation of immune complexes and reduces the risk of infection associated with fluid stasis.

Sensory Re-education

Sensory re-education is a type of cognitive behavior therapy with an aim to inhibit or stimulate sensory pathways. The neuropathic pain in burn survivors is thought to be resulted from complications or misperceptions of sensory experiences following damage to their peripheral nervous system. Thus, by using this therapy, the patients are reconditioned to recognize normal sensation. In a case series consisting of 17 patients who sustained neuropathic pain after burn injury, sensory re-education resulted in the improvement of the pain in 76% of patients.[53]

Others

Various therapies for chronic burn pain have been suggested in the literature, including hypnosis, yoga, virtual reality/augmented reality, deep breathing, and neuromodulation.[54,55] These modalities have demonstrated potential in reducing chronic pain and/or anxiety, offering the possibility of contributing to improved patient outcomes.

NERVE BLOCKS

In addition to their diagnostic utility, regional nerve blocks offer therapeutic benefits by providing temporary or long-term pain relief. Temporary blocks involve the injection of local anesthetics around specific nerves or nerve plexuses to prevent the transmission of pain signals to the brain.[42,56–58] Commonly used medications include lidocaine, ropivacaine, and bupivacaine, with the first two having a more rapid onset of action, while bupivacaine has a longer therapeutic duration.[59] The analgesic effects of temporary blocks typically last from hours to days and are commonly used to manage acute burn pain, effectively reducing the opioid requirement.[42,56] Although their use in chronic burn pain management is not well-established, temporary blocks have been effectively used for chronic pain from various conditions, including neuropathic-type pain.[57,58,60] An advantage of regional blocks is that they provide targeted pain relief with higher drug concentrations and fewer risks of systemic adverse effects compared with systemic medications. Long-term blocks can be achieved through nonsurgical or surgical means. The former involves agents such as alcohol, phenol, thermal, or electrical agents to induce damage to the neuronal pathway, while the latter involves surgically removing or selectively damaging certain areas of the nerve.[61–63]

In patients with CNP, nerve blocks can serve as an adjunct to provide longer-lasting pain relief. The choice of block placement depends on the suspected injured nerves. For the upper extremity, brachial plexus blocks can be considered, with interscalene blocks providing relief for the shoulder/upper arm region, and supraclavicular, infraclavicular, and axillary blocks offering relief for the hand.[56,57] Similarly, for lower extremity pain, lumbar plexus, sciatic, lateral femoral cutaneous, fascia iliaca, and saphenous blocks can be considered, while for truncal/abdominal pain, thoracic epidural, paravertebral, and intercostal blocks may be considered.[56,57]

SURGICAL INTERVENTIONS

In general, patients with burn-related CNP are initially managed with multimodal pharmacotherapy and medical therapies. If medical management proves ineffective, patients are evaluated for surgical intervention. A detailed physical examination or diagnostic nerve block can help assess whether there is an anatomic cause of peripheral neuropathy amenable to surgical treatment. Typically, pain resulting from mononeuropathy or mononeuropathy multiplex may benefit from surgical treatment since this type of nerve pain is secondary to end-neuromas, neuromas in continuity, scar-tethered nerves, or nerve compression.[64] Notably, if the patient can massage the painful area, surgery is relatively contraindicated unless motor dysfunction is present.[65] Once a patient is identified as a surgical candidate with, the following interventions can be considered.

Laser

Laser therapy has been established as an effective treatment for hypertrophic burn scars, improving not only scar appearance but also neuropathic pain.[19,66–68] This method works by delivering focused light energy to the skin that is absorbed by targeted components (chromophores), and inducing various photochemical/photothermal effects and subsequent cellular responses. The selective absorption of laser light by chromophores is determined by the wavelength and pulse duration, which can be manipulated by different laser devices.[69] Once photons are absorbed by the targeted chromophores in the skin such as hemoglobin, oxyhemoglobin, melanin, water, or collagen, they generate heat, and selectively affecting capillaries, pigmentation, and scar tissue.[70]

A deep dive into each laser option is beyond the scope of this article. In general, lasers can be categorized into ablative/nonablative, fractional/nonfractional, and vascular/non-vascular based on the target and mechanism of actions.[19,67,69] Ablative lasers promote collagen remodeling of the skin through its ablative action on the dermal and epidermal layers. In contrast, nonablative lasers induce damage to the dermis only without affecting the epidermis, resulting in less superficial damage and shorter recovery. Nonfractional lasers act on the entire projected surface area of the treated skin, whereas fractional lasers target only a

percentage of the projected area that is equally distributed. As such, the surrounding unaffected tissue with fractional laser treatment acts as a source of viability and contributes to collagen remodeling.[19] Lastly, vascular laser targets vessels beneath the epidermis and induce vessel destruction.

Both the superficial and deep scars can contribute to nerve compression. Laser therapy allows for targeting both superficial and deep layers of the scar to smooth the cutaneous continuity and induce dermal remodeling of abnormal collagen.[68] This process releases the tension caused by scar contracture, thereby may contribute to reducing nerve compression. In the senior author's practice, laser therapy is offered to patients with CNP if a hypertrophic scar is present, if there is no positive Tinel's sign, if there are multiple positive Tinel's signs, or if the involved nerve cannot be localized. Notably, laser therapy can be considered in select cases of focal nerve compression if a hypertrophic scar is symptomatic or if patients experience symptoms such as banding and stiffness. Surgical techniques and specific pre-, peri-, and postoperative management using laser therapies in treating hypertrophic burn scar were documented previously,[71] and the same approach has been found effective in treating burn-related CNP in the senior author's practice. In short, laser treatment should begin no sooner than 4 to 6 months after burn injury/wound closure, and therapy should continue every 4 to 6 weeks until reaching a predetermined treatment endpoint. Different modalities are used for specific symptoms (**Table 1**) and include pulsed dye laser (PDL), ablative fractional CO_2 laser, intense pulsed light laser, and Alexandrite laser. In particular, with PDL, care must be taken with increasingly pigmented skin to avoid complications of blistering, hypopigmentation, and postinflammatory hyperpigmentation. Patients with Fitzpatrick skin types 4, 5, and 6 must be treated with lower fluence across more sessions to avoid overtreatment. Notably, topical anesthetic can be implemented for patients undergoing fractionated laser ablation of symptomatic burn scars for its benefits in decreasing pain and the need for IV opioids.[72] Lastly, another application of laser technology is laser-assisted drug delivery, particularly for topical steroids. This method involves creating channels from the skin surface into the mid-level dermis, enabling a predictable mode of drug delivery.

Fat Grafting

Fat grafting has been used to treat various types of scars given its mechanical and regenerative

Table 1
Types of laser therapy commonly used for hypertrophic burn scars

Type (Wavelength)	Target Signs/ Symptoms	Setting	Intraoperative End-Point
Pulsed Dye Laser (595 nm)	Hypervascularity (pruritus, erythema)	Fluence 5–11 J/cm^2, 1.5 msec pulse duration, 7–10 mm spot size, $\leq$ 30% overlap, 1–2 passes	Ecchymosis
Ablative, Fractional CO2 Laser (10,600 nm)	Thick, stiff scars with abnormal texture	Deep ablation: density 3%–15%, frequency 600 Hz, 15–60 mJ/ micropulse, 1 pass Superficial ablation: frequency 150 Hz, 70–90 mJ/micropulse, 1 pass	Fine capillary bleeding
Alexandrite Laser (755 nm)	Folliculitis	Aiming beam 543 nm, 12 mm spot size, fluence 12.5 J/cm^2, minimal overlap, 1–2 passes	Audible pop and a visible spark
Intense Pulsed Light (515–590 nm filter)	Dyschromia	Fluence 18–24 J/cm^2 (dependent on skin type and targeted structure)	Slight darkening with erythema

properties, improving both the scar appearance and pain.[73–75] The regenerative property of lipoaspirate stems from adipose-derived stem cells and various other cell types that produce growth factors, proteins, and cytokines. These elements induce neovascularization, immunomodulation, cellular remodeling, and adipogenesis, thereby improving the overall cutaneous quality.[76–78] Fat grafting exerts its mechanical effects by acting as a filler to restore and offer cushion within the scar tissue, that is known to be deficient in subcutaneous adipose tissue. Specifically with neuropathic pain, the reason that fat grafting improves pain is likely due to the release of tension on nerves within the scar through fibrotic tissue release during grafting, lipoaspirate offering cushion around nerve endings/neuromas, and the process of cellular remodeling and decrease chronic inflammation.[74,75,79] Fat grafting has been shown as a safe and effective method to improve burn-related CNP.[79]

In the senior author's practice, fat grafting to the burn scar is offered to patients with CNP who have failed pharmacologic, medical, and laser therapies: specifically, in patients that show no Tinel's signs or multiple Tinel's signs on the physical examination. Recurrent symptoms following nerve surgery can also be effectively managed with fat grafting. Notably, this method can be particularly effective in patients without a focal neuroma.

A typical set-up is shown in **Fig. 1**. To start, the amount of lipoaspirate needed is determined by the surface area of the scar in a 1:1 ratio (10 mL processed fat for 10 cm^2 scar). Common donor sites include flanks, periumbilical, and infraumbilical regions. Tumescent technique (1000 mL Ringer's lactate, 50 mL 1% lidocaine, and 1 ampule epinephrine 1:1000) is used to harvest fat from the donor site with 1-, 2-, or 3-mm multiple sideport, rounded cannulas. Lipoaspirate is then processed using any system based on the surgeon's comfort level (Coleman technique, cotton gauze rolling, and washing and filtration). The

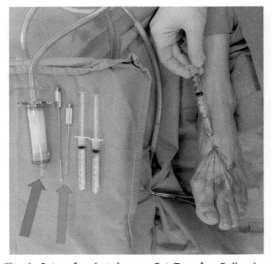

Fig. 1. Setup for Autologous Fat Transfer. Following the fat harvest, the LipiVage system (*red arrow*) was utilized for fat processing. Pickle fork, semi-sharp, and rounded cannula can be selected as they allow for scar release during injection (*blue arrow*).

senior author typically prefers the LipiVage system (Genesis Biosystems Inc, Lewisville, TX) because it is self-contained, protects fat graft from exposure to air, and allows small-volume graft transfer. Following fat graft processing, a flat- or rounded-single port cannula (<1 mm) is then used to inject processed fat directly under the scar, in a cross-hatched, radial, fanning pattern, at different subcutaneous tissue levels (Fig. 2). In this patient population, using microfat grafting is crucial to enhance graft survival, as the perforators may be lost due to burn injury, resulting in unpredictable and compromised vascularity. Rigotomy is performed as needed to help release scar tissue and allow for more fat tissue placement. Approximately 0.05 to 0.1 mL of fat was injected each time with the withdrawal of cannula, resulting in a final grafted fat volume of 0.5 to 1 mL per cm^2 of scar. Finally, the treated areas are dressed with xeroform, abdominal pads, Kerlix, and a loose ACE wrap for 5 days. If laser therapy was attempted first, fat grafting should be performed at a minimum of 1 month to allow the skin to recover. In general, patients are treated with 2 sessions of fat grafting, spaced 2 months apart. However, with previous laser treatment, selected patients may require only 1 session of fat grafting as laser therapy increases vascularity within the scars, resulting in better fat take. Notably, patients may experience an increase in pain immediately following surgery,

however, this typically resolves after 1 to 2 months.[79]

Nerve Decompression

Nerve decompression/release is performed to treat any focal area of nerve compression across the body caused by the burn scar. It has been demonstrated as effective, even when presented late after a burn injury, in improving pain, motor, and sensory functions, particularly in patients with electrical injuries.[10,15] Frequent locations for nerve compression include the carpal tunnel, Guyon's canal, cubital tunnel, tarsal tunnel, fibular head, and various other areas.[15] Candidates for nerve decompression include those who fail pharmacologic and medical therapies and exhibit anatomic focal areas of compression, with 1 to 2 positive Tinel's signs proximal to or within the burn scar. A positive EMG or NCV can be helpful but not required. Consideration may be given to releasing asymptomatic, nearby nerves if they are situated within or near the injury zone, or if the presence of surgical or burn scars would complicate a procedure at a later date. Oftentimes, patients may require more than 1 procedure with more than 1 nerve treated.[15] In addition to releasing scar bands and contractures and performing neurolysis (extraneural, perineural, or epineural with a firm intraneuronal scar) to relieve compressed nerves, modifications such as nerve

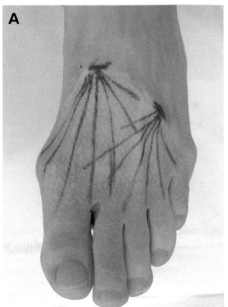 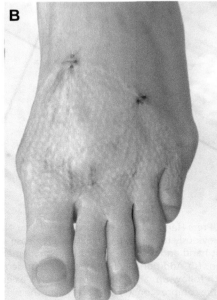

Fig. 2. Pre- and Post-Fat Transfer to the Dorsal Foot Burn Scar. (A) Prior to fat transfer, injection paths were marked in a fanning pattern. (B) Approximately 0.1 to 0.5 mL of fat was injected each time with withdrawal of cannula, resulting in a final grafted fat volume of 0.5 to 1 mL per cm^2 of scar.

transposition and flap coverage can be implemented as needed (**Fig. 3**). In those patients whose symptoms persist following decompression, neurectomy may be considered.[10,80] Although an optimal timing for nerve decompression is not clearly defined, it should be performed in patients with motor involvement sooner rather than later. Prior to surgery, all positive sites of Tinel's sign are marked to help identify the site of entrapment. An oblique, oval, or zig-zag incision is marked over the entrapment site, depending on the anatomic location. The incision site is planned at the junction between the skin grafts and native skin to avoid transecting through the skin grafts. If there is a scar contracture, tissue rearrangement should be considered to provide tissue coverage and release tension.

Neuroma Excision

In patients with CNP refractory to pharmacotherapy, medical therapy, and laser treatment, the presence of a neuroma may be the pain generator, with surrounding scar tissue tethering cutaneous sensory nerves. Although there is a lack of studies investigating the role of neuroma excision in burn-related CNP, neuroma excision is a known, definitive method to alleviate neuroma associated pain.[15,64,81,82] End-neuromas are usually attached to the burn scar from the deep side or can be within the burn scar.[83,84] Several treatment modifications have been proposed including excision only, excision with proximal stump relocation, and nerve loop with silicon sheath, all offering adequate pain relief.[15] Small neuromas in continuity are managed by the same surgical

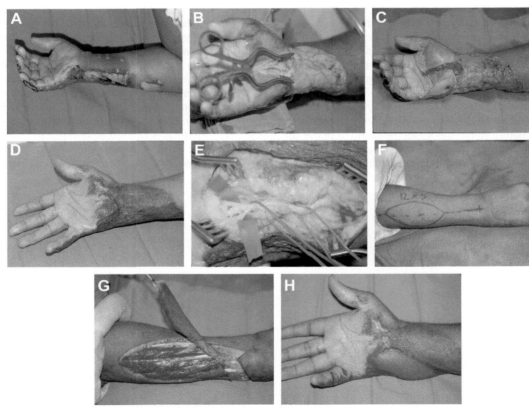

Fig. 3. Hot-Press Hand Burns with Secondary Ulnar Nerve Entrapment. (*A*) A patient with rheumatoid arthritis, who had previously undergone carpal tunnel release and extended synovectomy, presented with hot-press burns to the right hand and forearm. (*B*) Initial management included carpal tunnel release to address median nerve compression. (*C*) Additionally, burn wound debridement and fasciotomy of the hand were performed. (*D*) At the 6-month follow-up, all wounds were healed as expected, but the patient began to demonstrate symptoms of ulnar nerve compression. (*E*) Burn scars over the symptomatic site were excised, and ulnar nerve decompression of Guyon's canal was performed (ulnar nerve identified with vessel loops). (*F*) A posterior interosseous flap measuring 12 cm × 5 cm was designed to provide additional tissue coverage for the compression site. (*G*) The flap was elevated and rotated to cover lateral wrist and palm. (*H*) The patient experienced an uneventful postoperative course and successful relief of symptoms.

approach as end-neuromas. However, neurolysis or repair following resection should be considered in cases of large neuromas in continuity and scar-tethered nerve.[64,85] Other adjunctive techniques using flaps to provide coverage at the surgical site may be beneficial based on individual cases.[64,86]

In our experience, in selected patients with a verified Tinel's sign at the site of CNP, excision of the scar and any associated nerve tethering and neuroma can provide lasting, significant benefit. Candidates for neuroma excision are those who exhibit 1 to 2 positive Tinel's signs that are located at/under the burn scar. Prior to surgery, the location of the burn scar pain is evaluated with Tinel's sign, as this clinical sign not only suggests neuroma formation, but also provides an identifiable target for excision. Once the sites of Tinel's signs are marked, they are injected with 1 mL of 1% lidocaine with 1:100,000 epinephrine. If patients experience relief of their neuropathic burn pain, then we expect that they will improve with excision and schedule them for surgery. On the day of surgery, we repeat the marking of all positive sites of Tinel's sign, and a small ellipse is drawn to encompass the marked areas. The burn scar is then incised, dissecting it from distal to proximal under loupe magnification. In nearly all cases, a nerve or small nerve branch would be identified; this is traced proximally until reaching a healthy nerve (**Fig. 4**). An adequate length should be dissected to allow for the burial of the nerve. Next, the burn scar is excised, and the tethered nerve is transected. The cut end can either be buried in a subfascial or intramuscular fashion, or be managed with newer techniques such as targeted muscle reinnervation (TMR), regenerative peripheral nerve interface (RPNI), or VDMT

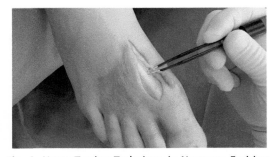

Fig. 4. Nerve Tracing Technique in Neuroma Excision. A small ellipse cut was made over the sites of Tinel's signs, and dissection was performed starting distally. Once a nerve was identified, it was traced proximally until reaching a healthy nerve. The distal neuroma was excised, and the proximal stump was transposed to a subfascial plane.

(Vascularized Denervated Muscle Targets), which are discussed in the corresponding section. Lastly, the defect is then closed; typically, due to laser treatment and fat grafting, the burn scar is supple enough to be closed primarily, even after excision of the overlying tissue (**Fig. 5**). In our experience, there still exists a role for the traditional approach of transposing the cut nerve end subfascially, into innervated muscle, or even bone, especially in situations whereby local muscle is limited. In such cases, although neuromas may reform, they tend to be less symptomatic, possibly due to their deeper location, resulting in less irritation.

Nerve Transfer

Within the recent decade, nerve procedures such as TMR, RPNI, and VDMT have rapidly evolved and gained popularity for their utility in nerve pain management.[87–90] These techniques focus on creating new interfaces between the damaged nerve and a designated target, promoting organized axon growth. Candidates for these nerve procedures are those with CNP refractory to other surgical interventions.

Targeted muscle reinnervation was initially developed to enhance myoelectric prosthesis control, with the discovery of pain relief as a secondary benefit, leading to the reapplication of TMR for the management and prevention of neuroma.[89,90] This method entails coapting the cut sensory/mixed nerve with a nearby motor nerve branch, allowing axons to regenerate into the muscle branches and reinnervate associated receptors, preventing neuroma formation. These principles can be applied for the treatment of symptomatic neuromas in mixed nerves or sensory nerves throughout the body,[91] as well as expanding to other treatment procedures for postmastectomy pain, migraine, and chronic abdominal pain.[31,92,93] Notably, since TMR involves the sacrifice of motor branches, it should be used with caution in the areas of the body with limited expendable muscles, particularly in distal extremities. A preoperative workup is similar to that discussed previously for neuroma excision. The plan for neuroma excision involves positioning the damaged sensory nerve's distal end near an expendable motor nerve branch of a nearby functional muscle. After identifying the motor nerve to the target muscle and confirming it with a nerve stimulator, dissection proceeds distally into the muscle until it branches to a minimal area of innervation, minimizing the denervation of muscle tissue. The proximal end of this motor branch is then severed, and coaptation is performed by connecting the distal part of the sensory nerve to the motor branch anchored into the target muscle, away from any weight-bearing surfaces.

Similar to TMR, RPNI provides a distal denervated muscle target for the regeneration of the damaged sensory nerve.[90,94] Unlike TMR, this technique does not require nerve coaptation but a transfer of a free nerve end into a free muscle graft. In contrast to the traditional bury-in-muscle technique, whereby the injured nerve end is placed within nearby innervated muscles, RPNI features unoccupied motor endplates that facilitate axonal ingrowth.[95] RPNI surgery has been shown to be effective in treating and preventing neuroma pain.[90,94,96] Preoperative workup for RPNI mirrors that of TMR, involving the assessment of suspected neuroma with Tinel's signs and possible diagnostic nerve block. Once the neuroma is identified and excised, a muscle graft is harvested from a healthy, expendable muscle.[94,96] The previously transected nerve ending is then placed in the middle of the graft in parallel to the muscle fibers with the distal nerve ending secured in place with nonabsorbable sutures. The muscle graft is wrapped around the nerve end entirely and secured with additional sutures. Next, the RPNI is buried within the surrounding soft tissue while ensuring the tensionless placement, deep away from weight-bearing surfaces. If the damaged nerve is of a larger caliber, it should be neurolyzed into individual fascicles, with each fascicle wrapped in a muscle graft.[96] This ensures that each graft remains relatively small, reducing the chances of necrosis and graft loss.

Lastly, VDMT is a recently developed technique that, similar to TMR and RPNI, provides a distal denervated target for axon regeneration from the damaged sensory nerve.[88] However, in contrast to RPNI which uses free muscle grafts, VDMT involves raising an island muscle flap on a pedicle in close proximity to the damaged sensory nerve end. The preserved blood supply to the muscle target allows the VDMT muscle flap to be larger than RPNI.[97,98] However, the dimension of a given VDMT is still limited by the orientation and amount of perfusion provided by its vascular pedicle. The optimal ratio of muscle volume to incoming axons to prevent neuroma formation is currently not defined.[88] Similar to TMR and RPNI, VDMT has been used to prevent and treat neuroma.[88,97] A detailed operative steps were described by Calotta and colleagues.[98] In the senior author's practice, VDMT is typically preferred in burn patients because of the alteration of regional blood supply and destruction of perforators in this patient population (**Fig. 6**). With this technique, muscle tissue is ensured to be vascularized by its pedicle, reducing the possibility of muscle loss. The sites of VDMT are then transposed to deeper tissue, away from the repeated pressure at the initial site.

TREATMENT ALGORITHM

We present our treatment algorithm as follows (**Fig. 7**): If motor symptoms are present, direct surgical management with nerve decompression should be considered promptly. Laser therapy is generally offered to all patients presenting with hypertrophic scars. Tinel's test is recommended in all patients. If Tinel's sign is absent, multiple, or if it cannot help localize a nerve, laser treatment is attempted. If 1 to 2 positive Tinel's signs are identified proximal to the symptomatic burn scar, nerve decompression is performed. If 1 to 2 positive Tinel's signs are identified over the symptomatic burn scar, both nerve decompression and neuroma with burn scar excision can be performed. If pain persists after laser therapy,

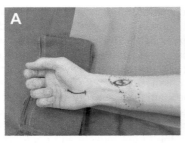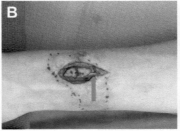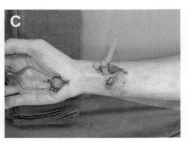

Fig. 5. Neuroma Excision and Nerve Release in Burn Scars. (*A*) An area of burn scars was dotted over the distal forearm, and a small ellipse was marked over the suspected neuroma site (sites of Tinel's signs). (*B*) Dissection was performed down to the fascia, and the lateral antebrachial cutaneous nerve (*red arrow*) was identified and traced proximally until reaching the normal segment. (*C*) Neuroma excision was performed distal to the identified normal segment. Additionally, a branch of an intact radial nerve was found tethered to the surrounding scar tissue and was released (*green arrow*).

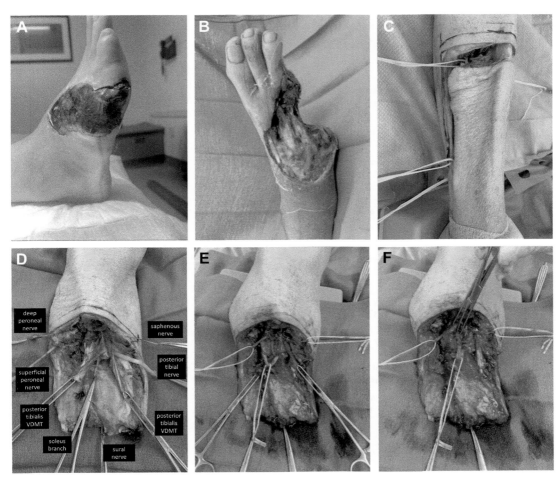

Fig. 6. Below-Knee Amputation with Vascularized Denervated Muscle Targets for Right Foot Burn Injury. (*A*) The patient presented with a full-thickness, 4th-degree burn on the right foot. (*B*) The foot was deemed unsalvageable following debridement. (*C*) One-stage approach for below-knee amputation in conjunction with VDMT was planned, with the goal of identifying as many nerves as possible to optimize flap options. (*D*) The posterior tibialis muscle was used to create two VDMT. The muscle was denervated while preserving its vascularity and leaving it attached to some of its tendon. (*E*) The tourniquet was released to check for bleeding. (*F*) The VDMT were transposed on themselves once released, and the distal skin flap was thinned out and closed. VDMT, vascularized denervated muscle targets.

nerve decompression, or neuroma excision, fat grafting is considered. If fat grafting is ineffective, nerve transfer procedures (TMR, RPNI, VDMT) can be offered to patients.

Managing patient expectations plays a pivotal role in long-term recovery and medical compliance. Prior to surgery, education should be provided regarding the natural evolution of CNP, including the possibility of spontaneous clinical improvement without surgery.[27,34] Understanding postoperative outcomes is essential, and surgical success can be measured by any metrics, whether subjective or objective. Frequently, success is associated with a definitive or moderate improvement in symptoms, improved motor functions, and/or a decreased need for a pharmacologic regimen.[15] Unsuccessful surgery, or the failure to alleviate pain, is considered a significant complication, often resulting from inappropriate patient selection or inefficiencies in the chosen surgical technique.[96] Recognizing and communicating these expectations establishes the foundation for a collaborative and informed decision-making process between the surgeon and patients. This patient-centric approach is crucial for effectively managing burn-related CNP, ensuring a comprehensive and supportive continuum of care.

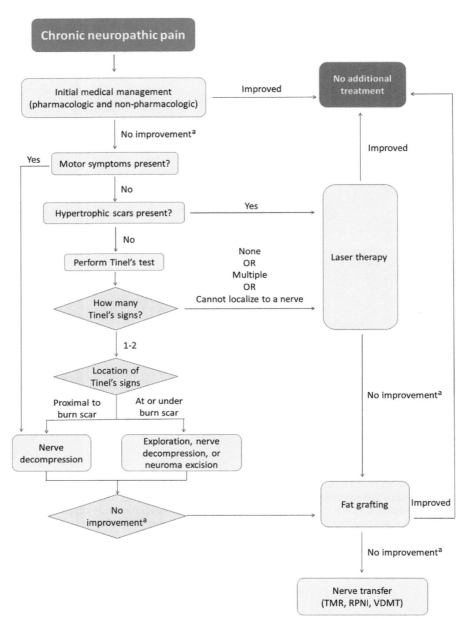

Fig. 7. Algorithm of surgical treatment for burn-related chronic neuropathic pain. If motor symptoms are present, direct surgical management with nerve decompression should be considered promptly. Laser therapy is generally offered to all patients presenting with hypertrophic scars. Tinel's test is recommended in all patients. If Tinel's sign is absent, multiple, or if it cannot help localize a nerve, laser treatment is attempted. If 1 to 2 positive Tinel's signs are identified proximal to the symptomatic burn scar, nerve decompression is performed. If 1 to 2 positive Tinel's signs are identified over the symptomatic burn scar, both nerve decompression and neuroma with burn scar excision can be performed. If pain persists after laser therapy, nerve decompression, or neuroma excision, fat grafting is considered. If fat grafting is ineffective, nerve transfer procedures can be offered to patients. RPNI, regenerative peripheral nerve interface; TMR, targeted muscle reinnervation; VDMT, vascularized denervated muscle targets. [a]Includes symptom plateau for ≥3 months.

CLINICS CARE POINTS

- While all patients should undergo a trial of pharmacologic and medical therapies, surgeons should diligently search for an anatomic cause of pain if these methods prove ineffective.
- Effective surgical management requires knowledge of neuropathic pain, recognition of surgical candidates, identification of the target symptoms, and proficiency in different techniques.
- Establishing a treatment team to manage pain through multidisciplinary therapies and guiding patients for appropriate expectations are paramount to long-term recovery outcomes.

DISCLOSURE

This research did not receive any specific grant from funding agencies in the public, commercial, or not-for-profit sectors.

REFERENCES

1. Klifto KM, Yesantharao PS, Lifchez SD, et al. Chronic nerve pain after burn injury: an anatomical approach and the Development and validation of a model to predict a patient's risk. Plast Reconstr Surg 2021; 148(4):548e–57e.
2. Klifto KM, Dellon AL, Hultman CS. Prevalence and associated predictors for patients developing chronic neuropathic pain following burns. Burns & Trauma 2020;8. tkaa011.
3. Klifto KM, Hultman CS, Dellon AL. Nerve pain after burn injury: a proposed Etiology-based classification. Plast Reconstr Surg 2021;147(3):635–44.
4. Gilron I, Baron R, Jensen T. Neuropathic pain: principles of diagnosis and treatment. Mayo Clin Proc 2015;90(4):532–45.
5. Woolf CJ, American College of Physicians. American Physiological Society. Pain: moving from symptom control toward mechanism-specific pharmacologic management. Ann Intern Med 2004;140(6):441–51.
6. Klifto KM, Yesantharao PS, Dellon AL, et al. Chronic neuropathic pain following hand burns: Etiology, treatment, and long-term outcomes. J Hand Surg Am 2021;46(1):67.e1-.e9.
7. Anastakis DJ, Peters WJ, Lee KC. Severe peripheral burn polyneuropathy: a case report. Burns Incl Therm Inj 1987;13(3):232–5.
8. Strong AL, Agarwal S, Cederna PS, et al. Peripheral neuropathy and nerve compression Syndromes in burns. Clin Plast Surg 2017;44(4):793–803.
9. Lippin Y, Shvoron A, Yaffe B, et al. Postburn peroneal nerve palsy–a report of two consecutive cases. Burns 1993;19(3):246–8.
10. Wu C, Calvert CT, Cairns BA, et al. Lower extremity nerve decompression in burn patients. Ann Plast Surg 2013;70(5):563–7.
11. Tsionos I, Leclercq C, Rochet JM. Heterotopic ossification of the elbow in patients with burns. Results after early excision. J Bone Joint Surg Br 2004; 86(3):396–403.
12. Salisbury RE, Dingeldein GP. Peripheral nerve complications following burn injury. Clin Orthop Relat Res 1982;163:92–7.
13. Marquez S, Turley JJE, Peters WJ. Neuropathy in burn patients. Brain 1993;116(2):471–83.
14. Khedr EM, Khedr T, El-Oteify MA, et al. Peripheral neuropathy in burn patients. Burns 1997;23(7): 579–83.
15. Rapolti M, Wu C, Schuth OA, et al. Under pressure: Applying practice-based Learning and improvement to the treatment of chronic neuropathic pain in patients with burns. Clin Plast Surg 2017;44(4): 925–34.
16. Henderson B, Koepke GH, Feller I. Peripheral polyneuropathy among patients with burns. Arch Phys Med Rehabil 1971;52(4):149–51.
17. Margherita AJ, Robinson LR, Heimbach DM, et al. Burn-associated peripheral polyneuropathy. A search for causative factors. Am J Phys Med Rehabil 1995;74(1):28–32.
18. Chan Q, Ng K, Vandervord J. Critical illness polyneuropathy in patients with major burn injuries. Eplasty 2010;10:e68.
19. Issler-Fisher AC, Waibel JS, Donelan MB. Laser modulation of hypertrophic scars: technique and practice. Clin Plast Surg 2017;44(4):757–66.
20. Henderson J, Terenghi G, McGrouther DA, et al. The reinnervation pattern of wounds and scars may explain their sensory symptoms. J Plast Reconstr Aesthet Surg 2006;59(9):942–50.
21. Browne AL, Andrews R, Schug SA, et al. Persistent pain outcomes and patient Satisfaction with pain management after burn injury. Clin J Pain 2011; 27(2):136.
22. Dauber A, Osgood PF, Breslau AJ, et al. Chronic persistent pain after severe burns: a Survey of 358 burn survivors. Pain Med 2002;3(1):6–17.
23. Malenfant A, Forget R, Papillon J, et al. Prevalence and characteristics of chronic sensory problems in burn patients. Pain 1996;67(2):493.
24. Choinière M, Melzack R, Papillon J. Pain and paresthesia in patients with healed burns: an exploratory study. J Pain Symptom Manage 1991;6(7):437–44.

25. Stanton E, Kowalske K, Won P, et al. Neuropathic pain after burn injury: a severe and common Problem in recovery. Ann Surg 2023. https://doi.org/10.1097/SLA.0000000000006146.

26. Van Loey NEE, de Jong AEE, Hofland HWC, et al. Role of burn severity and posttraumatic stress symptoms in the co-occurrence of itch and neuropathic pain after burns: a longitudinal study. Front Med 2022;9:997183.

27. Schneider JC, Harris NL, El Shami A, et al. A descriptive review of neuropathic-like pain after burn injury. J Burn Care Res 2006;27(4):524–8.

28. Colloca L, Ludman T, Bouhassira D, et al. Neuropathic pain. Nat Rev Dis Primers 2017;3:17002.

29. Nelson S, Conroy C, Logan D. The biopsychosocial model of pain in the context of pediatric burn injuries. Eur J Pain 2019;23(3):421–34.

30. Klifto KM, Dellon AL, Hultman CS. Risk factors associated with the progression from acute to chronic neuropathic pain after burn-related injuries. Ann Plast Surg 2020;84(6S):S382.

31. Caragher SP, Khouri KS, Raasveld FV, et al. The peripheral nerve Surgeon's role in the management of neuropathic pain. Plast Reconstr Surg Glob Open 2023;11(5):e5005.

32. Lifchez SD, Means KR, Dunn RE, et al. Intra- and Inter-Examiner Variability in performing Tinel's test. J Hand Surg 2010;35(2):212–6.

33. Decrouy-Duruz V, Christen T, Raffoul W. Evaluation of surgical treatment for neuropathic pain from neuroma in patients with injured peripheral nerves. J Neurosurg 2018;128(4):1235–40.

34. Gabriel V, Kowalske KJ, Holavanahalli RK. Assessment of recovery from burn related neuropathy by electrodiagnostic testing. J Burn Care Res 2009;30(4):668–74.

35. Arnold DMJ, Wilkens SC, Coert JH, et al. Diagnostic Criteria for symptomatic neuroma. Ann Plast Surg 2019;82(4):420.

36. Kollmer J, Bendszus M, Pham M, et al. Diagnostic Imaging in the PNS. Clin Neuroradiol 2015;25(2):283–9.

37. Chang KV, Mezian K, Naňka O, et al. Ultrasound Imaging for the cutaneous nerves of the extremities and relevant entrapment Syndromes: from anatomy to clinical implications. J Clin Med 2018;7(11):457.

38. Hjermstad MJ, Fayers PM, Haugen DF, et al. Studies comparing Numerical rating Scales, Verbal rating Scales, and Visual Analogue Scales for assessment of pain Intensity in Adults: a systematic literature review. J Pain Symptom Manag 2011;41(6):1073–93.

39. Klifto KM, Hultman CS. Pain management in burn patients: pharmacologic management of acute and chronic pain. Clin Plast Surg 2023. https://doi.org/10.1016/j.cps.2023.11.004.

40. Zor F, Ozturk S, Bilgin F, et al. Pain relief during dressing changes of major adult burns: Ideal analgesic combination with ketamine. Burns 2010;36(4):501–5.

41. Wasiak J, Spinks A, Costello V, et al. Adjuvant use of intravenous lidocaine for procedural burn pain relief: a randomized double-blind, placebo-controlled, cross-over trial. Burns 2011;37(6):951–7.

42. Abdelrahman I, Steinvall I, Elmasry M, et al. Lidocaine infusion has a 25% opioid-sparing effect on background pain after burns: a prospective, randomised, double-blind, controlled trial. Burns 2020;46(2):465–71.

43. Carr AC, McCall C. The role of vitamin C in the treatment of pain: new insights. J Transl Med 2017;15:77.

44. Niesters M, Martini C, Dahan A. Ketamine for chronic pain: risks and benefits. Br J Clin Pharmacol 2014;77(2):357–67.

45. Hupert C, Yacoub M, Turgeon LR. Effect of hydroxyzine on morphine analgesia for the treatment of postoperative pain. Anesth Analg 1980;59(9):690–6.

46. Souza JB de, Carqueja CL, Baptista AF. Physical rehabilitation to treat neuropathic pain. Rev dor 2016;17:85–90.

47. Lagueux É, Dépelteau A, Masse J. Occupational Therapy's Unique contribution to chronic pain management: a scoping review. Pain Res Manag 2018;2018:5378451.

48. Monstrey S, Middelkoop E, Vranckx JJ, et al. Updated scar management practical Guidelines: non-invasive and invasive measures. J Plast Reconstr Aesthetic Surg 2014;67(8):1017–25.

49. Momeni M, Hafezi F, Rahbar H, et al. Effects of silicone gel on burn scars. Burns 2009;35(1):70–4.

50. Goutos I, Ogawa R. Steroid tape: a promising adjunct to scar management. Scars Burn Heal 2017;3. 2059513117690937.

51. Atiyeh BS, El Khatib AM, Dibo SA. Pressure garment therapy (PGT) of burn scars: evidence-based efficacy. Ann Burns Fire Disasters 2013;26(4):205–12.

52. Loskotová A, Loskotová J, Suchanek I, et al. Myofascial-manual lymphatic drainage for burn trauma: a service evaluation. Br J Community Nurs 2017;22(Sup5):S6–12.

53. Nedelec B, Calva V, Chouinard A, et al. Somatosensory rehabilitation for neuropathic pain in burn survivors: a case series. J Burn Care Res 2016;37(1):e37–46.

54. Lee SY, hyun Park C, Cho YS, et al. Scrambler therapy for chronic pain after burns and its effect on the Cerebral pain Network: a prospective, double-Blinded, randomized controlled trial. J Clin Med 2022;11(15):4255.

55. Gasteratos K, Papakonstantinou M, Man A, et al. Adjunctive Nonpharmacologic interventions for the management of burn pain: a systematic review. Plast Reconstr Surg 2022;149(5):985e–94e.

56. Wardhan R, Fahy BG. Regional Anesthesia and acute pain management for adult patients with burns. J Burn Care Res 2023;44(4):791–9.

57. Hayek SM, Shah A. Nerve blocks for chronic pain. Neurosurg Clin N Am 2014;25(4):809–17.

58. De Cassai A, Geraldini F. Chronic pain and regional Anesthesia: a Call to action. J Clin Med 2023;12(5):1955.
59. Keramidas EG, Rodopoulou SG. Ropivacaine versus lidocaine in Digital nerve blocks: a prospective study. Plast Reconstr Surg 2007;119(7):2148.
60. De Cassai A, Bonanno C, Sandei L, et al. PECS II block is associated with lower incidence of chronic pain after breast surgery. Korean J Pain 2019;32(4):286–91.
61. Cappellari AM, Tiberio F, Alicandro G, et al. Intercostal neurolysis for the treatment of Postsurgical thoracic pain: a case series. Muscle Nerve 2018;58(5):671–5.
62. D'Souza RS, Hooten WM. Neurolytic blocks. Available at:. In: StatPearls. StatPearls Publishing; 2023 http://www.ncbi.nlm.nih.gov/books/NBK537360/. [Accessed 16 December 2023].
63. Choi EJ, Choi YM, Jang EJ, et al. Neural ablation and regeneration in pain practice. The Korean Journal of Pain 2016;29(1):3–11.
64. Elliot D. Surgical management of painful peripheral nerves. Clin Plast Surg 2014;41(3):589–613.
65. Vernadakis AJ, Koch H, Mackinnon SE. Management of neuromas. Clin Plast Surg 2003;30(2):247–68, vii.
66. Choi KJ, Williams EA, Pham CH, et al. Fractional CO2 laser treatment for burn scar improvement: a systematic review and meta-analysis. Burns 2021;47(2):259–69.
67. Klifto KM, Asif M, Hultman CS. Laser management of hypertrophic burn scars: a comprehensive review. Burns Trauma 2020;8:tkz002.
68. Hultman CS, Friedstat JS, Edkins RE, et al. Laser resurfacing and remodeling of hypertrophic burn scars: the results of a large, prospective, before-after cohort study, with long-term follow-up. Ann Surg 2014;260(3):519–29 [discussion: 529–32].
69. Patil UA, Dhami LD. Overview of lasers. Indian J Plast Surg 2008;41(Suppl):S101–13.
70. Anderson RR, Parrish JA. Selective photothermolysis: precise microsurgery by selective absorption of pulsed radiation. Science 1983;220(4596):524–7.
71. Hultman CS, Edkins RE, Wu C, et al. Prospective, before-after cohort study to assess the efficacy of laser therapy on hypertrophic burn scars. Ann Plast Surg 2013;70(5):521–6.
72. Edkins RE, Hultman CS, Collins P, et al. Improving comfort and throughput for patients undergoing fractionated laser ablation of symptomatic burn scars. Ann Plast Surg 2015;74(3):293–9.
73. Fredman R, Katz AJ, Hultman CS. Fat grafting for burn, Traumatic, and surgical scars. Clin Plast Surg 2017;44(4):781–91.
74. Brongo S, Nicoletti GF, La Padula S, et al. Use of lipofilling for the treatment of severe burn outcomes. Plast Reconstr Surg 2012;130(2):374e–6e.
75. Klinger M, Marazzi M, Vigo D, et al. Fat injection for cases of severe burn outcomes: a new perspective of scar remodeling and reduction. Aesthetic Plast Surg 2008;32(3):465–9.
76. Si Z, Wang X, Sun C, et al. Adipose-derived stem cells: Sources, potency, and implications for regenerative therapies. Biomed Pharmacother 2019;114:108765.
77. Brown JC, Shang H, Yang N, et al. Autologous fat transfer for scar prevention and remodeling: a randomized, Blinded, placebo-controlled trial. Plast Reconstr Surg Glob Open 2020;8(5):e2830.
78. Sultan SM, Barr JS, Butala P, et al. Fat grafting accelerates revascularisation and decreases fibrosis following thermal injury. J Plast Reconstr Aesthet Surg 2012;65(2):219–27.
79. Fredman R, Edkins RE, Hultman CS. Fat grafting for neuropathic pain after severe burns. Ann Plast Surg 2016;76(Suppl 4):S29–303.
80. Dobyns JH. Digital nerve compression. Hand Clin 1992;8(2):359–67.
81. Ferguson JS, Franco J, Pollack J, et al. Compression neuropathy: a late finding in the postburn population: a four-year institutional review. J Burn Care Res 2010;31(3):458–61.
82. Portilla AS, Bravo GL, Miraval FK, et al. A feasibility study assessing cortical plasticity in chronic neuropathic pain following burn injury. J Burn Care Res 2013;34(1):e48–52.
83. Ono T, Matsunaga W. Traumatic neuroma: multiple lesions in the Fingers Occurring after deep burns. J Dermatol 1990;17(12):760–3.
84. Mendonca DA, Staiano JJ, Drew PJ. An unusual cutaneous neuroma following a burn injury. J Plast Reconstr Aesthet Surg 2006;59(1):107.
85. Brogan DM, Kakar S. Management of neuromas of the upper extremity. Hand Clin 2013;29(3):409–20.
86. Kakinoki R, Ikeguchi R, Atiyya AN, et al. Treatment of posttraumatic painful neuromas at the digit tip using neurovascular island flaps. J Hand Surg Am 2008;33(3):348–52.
87. Eberlin KR, Ducic I. Surgical algorithm for neuroma management: a Changing treatment Paradigm. Plastic and Reconstructive Surgery – Global Open 2018;6(10):e1952.
88. Tuffaha SH, Glass C, Rosson G, et al. Vascularized, denervated muscle targets: a Novel approach to treat and prevent symptomatic neuromas. Plast Reconstr Surg Glob Open 2020;8(4):e2779.
89. Souza JM, Cheesborough JE, Ko JH, et al. Targeted muscle reinnervation: a Novel approach to Postamputation neuroma pain. Clin Orthop Relat Res 2014;472(10):2984.
90. Woo SL, Kung TA, Brown DL, et al. Regenerative peripheral nerve interfaces for the treatment of Postamputation neuroma pain: a Pilot study. Plast Reconstr Surg Glob Open 2016;4(12):e1038.

91. Janes LE, Fracol ME, Dumanian GA, et al. Targeted muscle reinnervation for the treatment of neuroma. Hand Clin 2021;37(3):345–59.

92. Chappell AG, Yang CS, Dumanian GA. Surgical treatment of abdominal Wall neuromas. Plast Reconstr Surg Glob Open 2021;9(5):e3585.

93. O'Brien AL, Kraft CT, Valerio IL, et al. Targeted muscle reinnervation following breast surgery: a Novel technique. Plast Reconstr Surg Glob Open 2020; 8(4):e2782.

94. Hooper RC, Cederna PS, Brown DL, et al. Regenerative peripheral nerve interfaces for the management of symptomatic hand and Digital neuromas. Plast Reconstr Surg Glob Open 2020; 8(6):e2792.

95. Bader D. Reinnervation of motor endplate-containing and motor endplate-less muscle grafts. Dev Biol 1980;77(2):315–27.

96. Kubiak CA, Kemp SWP, Cederna PS. Regenerative peripheral nerve interface for management of Postamputation neuroma. JAMA Surg 2018;153(7):681–2.

97. Suresh V, Schaefer EJ, Calotta NA, et al. Use of vascularized, denervated muscle targets for prevention and treatment of upper-extremity neuromas. J Hand Surg Glob Online 2023;5(1):92–6.

98. Calotta NA, Hanwright PJ, Giladi A, et al. Vascularized, denervated muscle targets for treatment of symptomatic neuromas in the upper extremity: Description of operative technique. Tech Hand Up Extrem Surg 2022;26(3):141–5.

Fat Grafting and Regenerative Medicine in Burn Care

Mario Alessandri Bonetti, MD[a], Nelson S. Piccolo, MD[b],
J. Peter Rubin, MD, MBA[a], Francesco M. Egro, MD, MSc, MRCS[a,c],*

KEYWORDS

• Burn care • Burn surgery • Regenerative medicine • Fat grafting • Fat transfer • Platelet rich plasma

KEY POINTS

• In acute burns, the application of fat grafting showed a decrease in length of hospital stay, less need for skin grafting, less contracture formation, and less hypertrophic scarring and demonstrated improved scar texture, with minimal risk of complications.
• In burn scars, the stem cell components delivered with fat grafting may exert a local paracrine effect to induce neovascularization and immunomodulation, which results in the formation of new blood vessels and fibrotic tissue and collagen deposition remodeling, improving the quality of the scar.
• Plasma-rich plasma (PRP) is an autologous material which can be used to treat a variety of medical conditions, acting as a transporter of growth factors (GFs) (platelet-derived growth factor [PDGF], transforming growth factor beta [TGF-b], vascular endothelial growth factor [VEGF], epidermal growth factor [EGF], insulin-like growth factor 1[IGF-1]) and other bioactive molecules which facilitate wound closure, improve angiogenesis, and reinforce re-epithelialization. PRP treatment could have the capability of accelerating burn wound healing without causing delaying in skin graft take and without the occurrence of any adverse reactions or infections, while improving the quality of the scar.
• Despite the promising results, most of the studies on regenerative treatments in burns are retrospective and small in size. For this reason, higher level evidence studies are necessary to objectively and predictively assess the real impact of fat grafting and PRP on acute burns and burn scars.

BACKGROUND

Burns are one of the most devastating injuries a person can suffer, and their treatment has been a medical challenge for centuries.[1] In clinical practice, deep burns require excision of the non-viable tissue and replace burned skin with viable tissue in a single or multiple stages. The most common reconstructive options include skin graft, dermal substitute, or flaps. For non-operative burns, various dressings are available, yet no ideal solution has been identified.[2] The sequelae associated with burn injuries are very severe, which may lead to significant functional, aesthetic, and psychosocial impairment.

In recent years, the use of biostimulants, GFs, and tissue-derived cell therapies is gaining more attention by the scientific community and research continues in an effort to find a treatment able to accelerate acute burn healing and able to prevent or reverse the abnormal scarring that often results from deep burns.

Regenerative therapies such as fat grafting and platelet-rich plasma (PRP) have emerged as new

---

[a] Department of Plastic Surgery, University of Pittsburgh Medical Center, Pittsburgh, PA, USA; [b] Division of Plastic Surgery, Pronto Socorro Para Queimaduras, Brazil; [c] Department of Surgery, University of Pittsburgh Medical Center, Pittsburgh, PA, USA
* Corresponding author. Department of Plastic Surgery, University of Pittsburgh Medical Center, 1350 Locust St, Medical Professional Building, Suite G103, Pittsburgh, PA 15219.
E-mail address: francescoegro@gmail.com

Clin Plastic Surg 51 (2024) 435–443
https://doi.org/10.1016/j.cps.2024.02.006
0094-1298/24/© 2024 Elsevier Inc. All rights reserved.

options in the armamentarium of plastic surgeons to tackle burn-related injuries and their long-term sequelae.[3,4]

FAT GRAFTING

The use of fat grafting has become increasingly popular in recent years due to several beneficial characteristics, including lack of immunogenicity, simple and safe surgical procedure, low cost, and easy accessibility. Fat grafting has been commonly used in both aesthetic and reconstructive surgery, such as facial contouring, breast augmentation, breast reconstruction, radiation-induced fibrosis, breast capsular contracture, post-traumatic deformities, congenital anomalies, and burn injuries.

Latest evidence posed increasing emphasis on not only the filling capability of adipose tissue but also on its regenerative capacity. Indeed, fat tissue consists of 2 main components: mature adipocyte cells and stromal vascular fraction (SVF).[5] SVF is composed of heterogeneous cell populations including adipose-derived stem cells (ADSC), endothelial precursor cells, pericytes, pre-adipocytes, endothelial cells, macrophages, lymphocytes, and other cells.[5–8] Although not fully understood, ADSCs may exert their beneficial effects via complex paracrine mechanisms. ADSCs likely stimulate and recruit other cells such as fibroblasts and keratinocytes through the secretion of a variety of GFs such as beta fibroblast growth factor (bFGF), keratinocyte growth factor (KGF), transforming growth factor beta (TGF-β), hepatocyte growth factor (HGF), and vascular endothelial growth factor (VEGF).[9] In vitro evidences show that hypoxia, lipopolysaccharide, and TNF-alpha are able to induce GFs release by ADSCs.[9] Their activity leads to neovascularization and immunomodulation, resulting in the neovascularization, remodeling of fibrotic tissue, and deposition of collagen, thereby potentially improving the quality of the scars.[10,11]

ADSCs are one of the forms of mesenchymal stem cells (MSCs) of adipose origin with an inherent property of self-renewal and multipotent differentiation.[12] Advantages of easy accessibility of the source, abundant availability, and fewer ethical concerns than bone marrow and embryonic stem cells render adipose-derived stem cells (ADSCs) suitable for use in regenerative medicine and tissue engineering.[13] ADSCs have been shown to play a role in antiaging and skin regeneration by forming tissue consisting of hypodermis, dermis, and epidermis.[14–16] It is this regenerative capacity that is of particular interest in burn wound

therapy, considering that deep burn wounds have limited potential to self-heal.

ADSCs display the capability of influencing a number of factors associated with the different phases of wound healing.[17] They can interact with immune system cells during the inflammatory phase supporting a more anti-inflammatory environment.[18] Their regenerative and angiogenic properties can interfere during the proliferative phase of the healing process through the secretion of pro-trophic and anti-apoptotic factors.[19] Eventually, ADSCs can influence the remodeling phase due to their ability to modulate and regulate the composition of the extracellular matrix.[20,21]

Fat Grafting in Acute Burns

Conventional burn wound management typically consists of skin grafting and/or regular dressing. However, dressing management can be a laborious and slow process, whereas skin grafting is associated with donor site morbidity, prolonged hospital stay, and often leading to contracture and unpleasant appearance of the scar.

Recently, there has been considerable progress in burn care and management, which has led to a rise in survival rates and functional status. Temporary skin substitutes, cultured epithelial autografts, stem cell therapy, and other treatments are viable alternatives to traditional dressings, and can improve the care of burn patients, even though they can be costly and should be used judiciously.

Adipose-based therapies have been suggested as a novel approach in acute burns to accelerate the healing process and enhance the long-term functioning and appearance of burn scars.

Most of the available knowledge on the use of ADSC in acute burns is derived from animal studies, which have supplied baseline scientific data and encouraged clinical studies. Animal studies confirmed that ADSC can significantly accelerate wound healing, particularly in second-degree burns.[22] However, clinical studies have recently begun to report on the effectiveness of adipose-based therapies in acute burns in humans.

Abouzaid and colleagues[23] performed a randomized control clinical (RCT) trial on 100 acute burn patients, in which they administered a single injection of autologous fat grafting processed via the Coleman technique at the level of the superficial subcutaneous layer in superficial and deep partial thickness burns, followed by topical administration of nanofat on the wound bed. Dressing with cryopreserved nanofat was performed averagely every 2 days. As a result, they observed a decrease in total hospital stay days, less need for further skin grafting, less contracture formation, less hypertrophic scarring, and improved scar texture. In their study, histologic analysis showed that the fat grafting group had a more rapid deposition of collagen in the first month and then the rate reached a plateau, whereas the control group demonstrated an increase in collagen deposition at 3 months post-intervention. The authors concluded that autologous fat grafting has demonstrated its potential to be a successful therapeutic option for burn wounds, as it can address both the tissue impairment and poor wound profile of burn injuries. Adipose-based therapies may be used in conjunction with other surgical techniques or as a stand-alone therapy.

Further evidence comes from Piccolo and colleagues,[24] who investigated the use of fat grafting, processed using the Coleman technique, in burn wounds at 3 weeks or more with no apparent progression to healing, and in subacute burn or other non-healing wounds within more than 6 weeks after the burn injury. The protocol employed involved repeated applications of fat grafting (every 2–4 weeks) deposited in several passes under the wound bed or applied locally over its entire surface until healing or a definitive procedure is planned (eg, wound closure, skin grafting, flap). They successfully treated 240 patients with burn or trauma wounds. They reported a minimal risk of complications associated with their protocol. They also observed marked improvement even in area of critical structure exposure such as bone.

Piccolo and colleagues[25] also evaluated the effectiveness of adipose tissue in the treatment of 27 patients suffering from facial acute burns. The fat harvested and processed using the Coleman technique was then infiltrated deep to the burn tissue. After the fat grafting procedure, debridement of non-vital tissues was completed and more adipose tissue was applied as a biological dressing over the wound, which was then covered by a petrolatum gauze. Averagely, 2.5 sessions were performed. Even in cases of bone exposure, the fat was delivered directly over the area. All the patients with superficial or deep partial thickness burns healed. The 8 cases of bone exposure eventually developed healthy granulation tissue and were ultimately skin grafted with success.

The understanding of the exact mechanisms related to the action of fat grafting in acute burns in human remains unclear. However, various clinical studies have demonstrated its benefits and further research is needed before the definitive introduction of fat grafting in acute burn patients' care.

Fat Grafting in Burn Scars

Several techniques have been described for treating scar resulting from burn injuries, including silicon sheet application, intralesional injection of corticosteroids, compression therapy, topical tamoxifen therapy, intralesional fluorouracil, and cryotherapy.[26–28] Still low level of evidence exists on the effectiveness of different types of lasers, such as intense pulse light or fractional nonablative laser, on scar improvement.[29] However, the lack of gold-standard therapy and the unconvincing efficacy of available options along with the impact of burn scars on social interactions and quality of life of burn patients stand at the base for further research on this topic.[30]

Burn scars often present as hypertrophic scars. Their incidence varies between 30% and 90% after a burn injury, depending on the severity and depth of the burn.[31] Hypertrophic scars result from the abnormal deposition and remodeling of the extracellular matrix and collagen fibers and appear raised, red, itchy, and painful sometimes.[31]

Interest in fat grafting for problematic scars has grown due to the recognition of the positive properties that transferred fat can have on quality of local tissue and any type of scars. The effect of fat grafting on scar quality is thought to be related to its inherent regenerative capacity. The stem cell components delivered with fat grafting may exert a local paracrine effect to induce neovascularization and immunomodulation, which results in the formation of new blood vessels and fibrotic tissue and collagen deposition remodeling, improving the quality of the scar. The available evidence supports the use of adipose tissue–based treatments as a minimal invasive and low-cost alternative to surgical scar revision able to alleviate scar rigidity, firmness, texture, and appearance. However, despite the increasing application of fat grafting in burn scars, consistent results and large RCTs are still missing.

Two case-control studies have been conducted using "split scar" methods, where one-half of the scar was injected with fat and the other half with saline. Bruno and colleagues[32] investigated the effects of fat grafting processed using the Coleman technique on 93 burn scar patients. They observed an improvement in scar quality in the areas that were injected with fat. Specifically, they noted improved vascularization of the dermal papillae, normal collagen fibers organization, improved pigmentation 6 months after lipofilling, and significant scar improvement based on the Vancouver Scar Scale (VSS).

Klinger and colleagues[33] published the largest series of 694 patients with problematic scars

(376 of which were burn-related) who underwent autologous fat grafting using the Coleman technique. In all patients, an improvement in scar quality was observed, particularly in terms of pain relief and increased elasticity. Twenty of these patients underwent a split scar assessment, evaluated using the Patient and Observer Scar Assessment Scale questionnaire and Durometer measurements. Those areas that had been fat grafted showed a significant decrease in hardness and an overall improvement in scar qualities except for itching.

Gargano and colleagues[34] prospectively enrolled 12 patients with persisting retracting burn scars already treated with scar release, skin grafts, or Z-plasties. All analyzed scars limited range of motion of the affected joints. The authors performed subcision (percutaneous release) of the scar cords combined with multiple sessions (max 3) of fat grafting under the treated area. The adipose tissue was first washed with ringer lactate and then processed on non-adherent gauze pads. In their cohort, all patients showed improvement in both scar quality according to the VSS and range of motion, assessed using a goniometer. The regenerative effect of fat grafting was measured using high-definition ultrasound and histology, which revealed an increased deposition of collagen I and regular orientation of the fibers as in mature healing dermis after the fat grafting.

Byrne and colleagues[35] conducted a retrospective study on 13 patients affected by hand burn scars and contractures, causing decreased range of motion and poor cosmesis. The authors performed a single session of needle subcision combined with fat grafting processed according to the Coleman technique. At a mean follow-up of 9.1 months, they observed a significant improvement in total active motion measured with a goniometer, Michigan Hand Questionnaire, and Patient Observer Scar Assessment Scale (POSAS). Specifically, according to the POSAS scale, the authors reported improvement in scar color, thickness, stiffness, and regularity. No significant difference was detected between pre-operative and post-operative disability of the arm, shoulder, and hand.

Erol and colleagues[27] conducted a retrospective study on 288 patients with hypertrophic scars resulting from burn injuries. Their treatment protocol consisted of multiple sessions of non-ablative fraction carbon laser combined with fat grafting processed using the Coleman technique. Improvement in the clinical appearance was measured using a 4-point Likert scale. The 95% of the patients rated the improvement 3 or 4 out of 4 at a mean follow-up of 3.6 years. The authors observed enhanced texture, softness, pliability, and color. They reported that the degree of improvement was variable and appeared to be related to the severity of the scar and the type of skin involved. In men with burns to facial hair-bearing areas, the combined treatment allowed the injured skin to become suitable for hair transplantation.

Xu and colleagues[36] reported the use of nanofat under and within hypertrophic burn scars in 80 patients. Each patient was treated 3 times with an interval of 3 months and was followed up to 3 years. The authors reported scar improvement in terms of texture, elasticity, and color in 84% of the cases. In 10%, they noticed some improvement, while no improvement was noted only in 6% of the patients. Histologic examination before and after treatment showed a significant decrease in collagen fiber density and a more neatly arrangement of the fibers. Their findings suggest the restorative and anti-fibrotic effect of fat grafting on hypertrophic burn scars.

Piccolo and colleagues[25] treated 84 patients affected by facial hypertrophic scarring from burn injuries with subcision and fat grafting processed using the Coleman technique. They performed up to 4 sessions of fat grafting for each patient. Piccolo and colleagues developed a protocol consisting of fat grafting, followed by dermabrasion by means of fractional carbon (CO_2) laser or microneedling with a derma-roller. Eventually, they applied fat grafting on the scar surface and then covered it with a petrolatum gauze and further dressing. The authors reported an increase in elasticity and malleability of the scar tissue as well as decrease in volume and thickness. They also reported that upon informing the patients about the proposed procedures (CO_2 laser or microneedling), most of them preferred microneedleing with a derma-roller, this way avoiding the temporary "skin wound" usually resulting from the fractional CO_2 laser abrasion.

Brongo and colleagues[37] performed lipofilling for hypertrophic scars in 18 burn patients. All patients showed improved aesthetic appearance and patient's satisfaction using a 10-point Likert scale. Histology tests at 12 months follow-up validated the clinical improvements in the scars. They observed signs of new collagen deposition, angiogenesis, and dermal hyperplasia in their scars, demonstrating the advantages of adipose tissue-based treatments.

The precise mechanism by which fat grafting might improve scars quality is still under investigation. Scars caused by trauma or burns often lack volume, especially in the subcutaneous layer, which can be remarkably deficient in severe burns. Adipose tissue has been considered as an ideal filler to restore volume, shape, and to provide cushioning and softness, allowing not only an improvement in scar appearance but also in symptoms and functionality.

Indeed, fat grafting has been also proposed as treatment for reducing burn scar neuropathic pain.[38–40]

Fredman and colleagues[39] showed alleviation of neuropathic pain in 7 patients with refractory neuropathy at the level of the burn scar despite pharmacologic regimens, laser modulation, and in some cases, previous surgical decompression. According to the Patient-Reported Outcomes Measurement Information System, the mean preoperative score dropped from 3.4 to 1.45 at 1-year follow-up. They suggested that fat grafting could potentially reduce neuropathic pain by forming a physical barrier around nerve endings. Release of fibrotic tissue occurs during grafting, and small deposits of fat are left in place, releasing tension on nerves within the scar. The stem cell components of the grafted adipose tissue might drive nerve repair and soft tissue healing in an uneventful fashion. However, the exact process is yet to be understood.

Despite the considerable enthusiasm regarding the use of fat grafting as a method to improve the aesthetics and function of burn scars, growing debate exists in the literature. Recent RCTs have shown an improvement in the structural quality of the scar but have failed to demonstrate a clear superiority of fat grafting compared to controls. However, it is important to take into account that although these studies have a high level of evidence, they present several limitations including the small sample size, the inclusion of scars that do not derive from burns, the use of only 1 session of fat grafting, and no clear indication for scar revision.

Gal and colleagues[41] randomized 8 pediatric burn scars into 2 halves: one was injected with autologous fat graft and the other with saline. The harvested fat was processed according to the Coleman technique. Similar improvement in scar appearance and pliability occurred in both the groups.

Brown and colleagues[37] conducted a study on 17 patients with scars of different etiology including burn treated. They compared scars treated with fat grafting to paired scars treated with saline as a control. Fat was processed with centrifugation at 1200 g for 3 minutes. They reported that autologous fat grafting improved the quality of the scar from both the patient and the observer perspective, but they did not find any difference from scar treated with saline in terms of color, scar elasticity, and histology.

The current literature on the use of fat grafting in burn scar includes mainly adipose tissue manipulated according to the Coleman technique. Investigations on the efficacy of other types of ADSC-based therapies in clinical studies are still missing.

There are several limitations in the available literature on fat grafting in burns. Firstly, only few studies were designed with a control group. Secondly, most of the studies lacked prospective collection of data. Thirdly, histology before and after surgery was rarely investigated. Additionally, most of the studies performed only 1 session of fat grafting, which could underestimate its effectiveness.

PLATELET-RICH PLASMA

Plasma-rich plasma (PRP) is an autologous material which can be used to treat a variety of medical conditions.[42]

Research has indicated that platelets contain several biologically active proteins, such as VEGF, PDGF, EGF, TGF-b, FGF, and IGF-1 and IGF-2.[43,44] These proteins can affect a range of cellular processes, like homing of stem cells, cellular migration, proliferation, differentiation, angiogenesis, macrophage activation, and synthesis of collagen and matrix. Owing to its low cost, easy and fast isolation, histocompatibility, and lack of major side effects, PRP has become an attractive option for use in regenerative medicine.[42,45]

There are different ways for obtaining PRP. Generally, whole blood is collected in a tube and mixed with an anti-coagulant. It is then centrifuged at a soft spin of 200 g for 15 minutes to isolate and remove the red blood cells (RBCs). Then, 3 layers are visible: an upper layer of pure platelet-rich plasma (P-PRP), leukocyte and PRP (L-PRP), pure platelet-rich fibrin (P-PRF), and leucocyte-rich and platelet-rich fibrin (L-PRF); an intermediate layer of white blood cells (WBCs); and a bottom layer of RBCs. RBCs are discarded. To achieve pure PRP (P-PRP), the upper layer and intermediate layer are transferred to another tube, and platelets are concentrated at a higher speed of centrifugation (hard spin of 400 g for 15 min) to form a soft pellet at the bottom. The supernatant, containing PPP (platelet-poor plasma) is then discarded and the remaining PRP is homogenized in 5 mL of PRP to increase concentration. Finally, calcium chloride or thrombin is used to activate the GFs, resulting in activated PRP.[42,46]

For more than 20 years, PRP has been used to treat a wide range of medical issues, such as traumatic wounds, ulcers, surgical wounds, tendinopathies, ostheoarthritis, and others.[42]

PRP acts as a transporter of GFs (PDGF, TGF-b, VEGF, EGF, IGF-1) and other molecules.[47] Despite still being debatable if the stimulatory effect of PRP on cells is due to compounds from platelets or high levels of GFs,[43] the release of numerous active substances at high concentrations has been observed. These substances, in turn, enhance healing in acute and chronic wounds by activating cellular migration and proliferation. PRP has been found to possess mitogenic and chemotactic properties on various cell types, such as fibroblasts, keratinocytes, and epithelial cells, which are found in wounds. It stimulates the local production of GFs and helps to facilitate wound closure, improve angiogenesis, and reinforce re-epithelialization.[43,47] Moreover, PRP has been reported to possibly suppress cytokine release and reduce inflammation, interacting with macrophages to improve tissue healing and regeneration. For these reasons, PRP could be a powerful tool in accelerating wound healing in burns.

It has been suggested that PRP in burns can lead to quicker hemostasis and tissue attachment due to the larger amount of normal modulators of regeneration, which may result in enhanced tissue regeneration, reduced pain, and less blood loss.[48] Several case reports or small series have been published in the literature on this topic, but only few well-designed studies have investigated the role of PRP in burns.

Maghsoudi and colleagues[49] conducted an RCT on 50 participants affected by second-degree or third-degree acute burns. They treated part of the wound with PRP and part with silver sulfadiazine, covered by an occlusive dressing. The majority (90%) in the PRP group achieved complete healing, compared to 38% in the sulfadiazine group. Also, the mean time to complete healing in the PRP group was 9.5 ± 4.6 days versus 12.2 ± 5.4 in the silver sulfadiazine group.

Marck and colleagues[50] conducted an RCT on 52 subjects with acute burns investigating the skin graft take with or without application of PRP on the wound bed before grafting. There was no statistically significant difference between the mean graft take rate nor between the mean epithelialization rate at day 5 to 7 between the PRP-treated and standard care areas. However, PRP-treated burns showed overall enhanced epithelialization compared to controls. Long-term results in scar appearance showed no statistically significant differences between PRP and standard-treated areas in POSAS scores of both the patients and observers, DermaSpectrometer scores, and Cutometer scores at 3, 6, and 12 months.

Dai and colleagues[51] conducted a case-control study on hypertrophic scars resulting from burn injury treated with application of ablative fractional carbon laser (AFCL) with or without PRP distributed onto the wound. Among the enrolled patients, 31 patients were treated with AFCL and PRP combined. The remaining 19 patients underwent AFCL only. Sessions were conducted every month for 6 consecutive sessions. All cases were evaluated by 2 blinded dermatologists using the University of North Carolina 4P Scar Scale (UNC4P) and the VSS. Both the groups experienced improvement in pliability, pain, pruritus and paraesthesia, thickness, and pigmentation scores. However, after combined treatment with AFCL and PRP, the UNC4P and VSS scores were significantly lower than those after AFCL treatment alone. The differences between the UNC4P and VSS scores at the third and sixth months were statistically significant. This suggests that the combined application of AFCL and PRP can improve scars more effectively.

Current literature has shown that PRP treatment could have the capability of accelerating burn wound healing without causing delaying in skin graft take and without the occurrence of any adverse reactions or infections, while improving the quality of the scar. Although the association of PRP and fat grafting has been proven beneficial in terms of fat graft resorption rate and ADSCs activity,[52,53] scarce evidence exists at present about their potential synergic application in burns, and it may represent an interesting direction for future studies. Lastly, although PRP is low cost, easy to use, and non-invasive, a paucity of knowledge in its application in burns remains. Also, burn patients have an altered systemic physiology, and platelet quantity and quality can affect PRP quality as well. Thus, further research is needed before its introduction.

SUMMARY

Burn scars have significant impact on patients' quality of life and function. Current studies appear to demonstrate a certain degree of improvement in scar quality and symptoms following autologous fat grafting.

Fat grafting and PRP have the potential to revolutionize the way burns are treated, offering a quicker recovery and more aesthetically pleasing results than conventional treatments.

Encouraging evidence on the beneficial effects of adipose-based therapies in acute burns and burn scars has been reported in the past year. Histologic studies have shown improvements in angiogenesis, collagen organization, and neuropathic pain. Human studies have shown similar biochemical effects in addition to improvements in clinical features such as skin texture, softness, coloration, and function. Less knowledge is available on the role of PRP compared to fat grafting as a treatment for burn injuries. However, PRP demonstrated safety, non-invasiveness, and positive properties in wound healing; therefore, further research on this topic is mandatory.

Despite the promising nature of current literature, majority of studies are retrospective and small in size. For this reason, higher level evidence with randomized, blinded, and placebo-controlled studies is necessary to objectively and predictively assess the real impact of fat grafting on burn scars. Furthermore, predictive factors of enhanced response should be identified in order to better define surgical indications. Nevertheless, there is substantial evidence that fat grafting is able to improve the healing process in acute burns and to remodel hypertrophic and dystrophic burn scars. Regenerative medicine has the prospect of playing a key role in the future of acute and reconstructive burn care. Fat grafting and PRP should be considered another useful tool in the armamentarium of the modern burn and reconstructive surgeon.

CLINICS CARE POINTS

- In acute burns, fat grafting is able to reduce the requirement for skin grafting, decrease the likelihood of contracture formation and hypertrophic scarring, and improve the scar texture.
- In burn scars, fat grafting promotes neovascularization and fibrotic tissue remodeling ultimately enhancing the overall quality of the scar.
- Platelet-rich plasma has the potential to enhance wound healing by accelerating stages including hemostasis and re-epithelization. It has beneficial effects also on the quality of chronic burn scar, and it can complement fat grafting procedures.

DISCLOSURE

The authors have no relevant commercial or financial conflicts of interest or funding sources.

REFERENCES

1. Smolle C, Cambiaso-Daniel J, Forbes AA, et al. Recent trends in burn epidemiology worldwide: a systematic review. Burns 2017;43(2):249–57.
2. Hermans MHE. Results of an internet survey on the treatment of partial thickness burns, full thickness burns, and donor sites. J Burn Care Res 2007; 28(6):835–47.
3. Sharma S, Muthu S, Jeyaraman M, et al. Translational products of adipose tissue-derived mesenchymal stem cells: Bench to bedside applications. World J Stem Cells 2021;13(10):1360–81.
4. Surowiecka A, Chrapusta A, Klimeczek-Chrapusta M, et al. Mesenchymal stem cells in burn wound management. Int J Mol Sci 2022;23(23):15339.
5. Gentile P, Scioli MG, Bielli A, et al. Concise review: the Use of adipose-derived stromal vascular fraction cells and platelet rich plasma in regenerative plastic surgery. Stem Cell 2017;35(1):117–34.
6. Bora P, Majumdar AS. Adipose tissue-derived stromal vascular fraction in regenerative medicine: a brief review on biology and translation. Stem Cell Res Ther 2017;8(1):145.
7. Zuk PA, Zhu M, Ashjian P, et al. Human adipose tissue is a source of multipotent stem cells. Mol Biol Cell 2002;13(12):4279–95.
8. Zuk PA, Zhu M, Mizuno H, et al. Multilineage cells from human adipose tissue: implications for cell-based therapies. Tissue Eng 2001;7(2):211–28.
9. Kim WS, Park BS, Sung JH. The wound-healing and antioxidant effects of adipose-derived stem cells. Expert Opin Biol Ther 2009;9(7):879–87.
10. Tonnard P, Verpaele A, Carvas M. Fat grafting for facial Rejuvenation with nanofat grafts. Clin Plast Surg 2020;47(1):53–62.
11. van Dongen JA, Langeveld M, van de Lande LS, et al. The effects of facial Lipografting on skin quality: a systematic review. Plast Reconstr Surg 2019; 144(5):784e–97e.
12. Seo Y, Shin TH, Kim HS. Current Strategies to enhance adipose stem cell function: an update. Int J Mol Sci 2019;20(15):3827.
13. Orbay H, Tobita M, Mizuno H. Mesenchymal stem cells isolated from adipose and other tissues: basic biological properties and clinical applications. Stem Cells Int 2012;2012:461718.
14. Spiekman M, Przybyt E, Plantinga JA, et al. Adipose tissue-derived stromal cells inhibit TGF-β1-induced differentiation of human dermal fibroblasts and keloid scar-derived fibroblasts in a paracrine fashion. Plast Reconstr Surg 2014;134(4):699–712.
15. Gaur M, Dobke M, Lunyak VV. Mesenchymal stem cells from adipose tissue in clinical applications for Dermatological indications and skin Aging. Int J Mol Sci 2017;18(1):208.
16. Nie C, Yang D, Xu J, et al. Locally administered adipose-derived stem cells accelerate wound healing through differentiation and vasculogenesis. Cell Transplant 2011;20(2):205–16.
17. Maranda EL, Rodriguez-Menocal L, Badiavas EV. Role of mesenchymal stem cells in dermal repair in

burns and diabetic wounds. Curr Stem Cell Res Ther 2017;12(1):61–70.

18. Li N, Hua J. Interactions between mesenchymal stem cells and the immune system. Cell Mol Life Sci 2017;74(13):2345–60.

19. Wu Y, Chen L, Scott PG, et al. Mesenchymal stem cells enhance wound healing through differentiation and angiogenesis. Stem Cell 2007;25(10):2648–59.

20. Riis S, Stensballe A, Emmersen J, et al. Mass spectrometry analysis of adipose-derived stem cells reveals a significant effect of hypoxia on pathways regulating extracellular matrix. Stem Cell Res Ther 2016;7(1):52.

21. Hyldig K, Riis S, Pennisi CP, et al. Implications of extracellular matrix production by adipose tissue-derived stem cells for Development of wound healing therapies. Int J Mol Sci 2017;18(6):1167.

22. Li Y, Xia WD, Van der Merwe L, et al. Efficacy of stem cell therapy for burn wounds: a systematic review and meta-analysis of preclinical studies. Stem Cell Res Ther 2020;11(1):322.

23. Abouzaid AM, El Mokadem ME, Aboubakr AK, et al. Effect of autologous fat transfer in acute burn wound management: a randomized controlled study. Burns 2022;48(6):1368–85.

24. Piccolo NS, Piccolo MS, Piccolo MTS. Fat grafting for treatment of burns, burn scars, and other difficult wounds. Clin Plast Surg 2015;42(2):263–83.

25. Piccolo NS, Piccolo MS, de Paula Piccolo N, et al. Fat grafting for treatment of facial burns and burn scars. Clin Plast Surg 2020;47(1):119–30.

26. Parry I, Sen S, Palmieri T, et al. Nonsurgical scar management of the face: does early versus late intervention affect outcome? J Burn Care Res 2013;34(5):569–75.

27. Onur Erol O, Agaoglu G, Jawad MA. Combined non-ablative laser and Microfat grafting for burn scar treatment. Aesthet Surg J 2019;39(4):NP55–67.

28. Sheng M, Chen Y, Li H, et al. The application of corticosteroids for pathological scar prevention and treatment: current review and update. Burns Trauma 2023;11. tkad009.

29. Leszczynski R, da Silva CA, Pinto ACPN, et al. Laser therapy for treating hypertrophic and keloid scars. Cochrane Database Syst Rev 2022;9(9):CD011642.

30. Chiang RS, Borovikova AA, King K, et al. Current concepts related to hypertrophic scarring in burn injuries. Wound Repair Regen 2016;24(3):466–77.

31. Niessen FB, Spauwen PH, Schalkwijk J, et al. On the nature of hypertrophic scars and keloids: a review. Plast Reconstr Surg 1999;104(5):1435–58.

32. Bruno A, Delli Santi G, Fasciani L, et al. Burn scar lipofilling: immunohistochemical and clinical outcomes. J Craniofac Surg 2013;24(5):1806–14.

33. Klinger M, Caviggioli F, Klinger FM, et al. Autologous fat graft in scar treatment. J Craniofac Surg 2013; 24(5):1610–5.

34. Gargano F, Schmidt S, Evangelista P, et al. Burn scar regeneration with the "SUFA" (Subcision and Fat Grafting) technique. A prospective clinical study. JPRAS Open 2018;17:5–8.

35. Byrne M, O'Donnell M, Fitzgerald L, et al. Early experience with fat grafting as an adjunct for secondary burn reconstruction in the hand: technique, hand function assessment and aesthetic outcomes. Burns 2016;42(2):356–65.

36. Xu X, Lai L, Zhang X, et al. Autologous chyle fat grafting for the treatment of hypertrophic scars and scar-related conditions. Stem Cell Res Ther 2018;9(1):64.

37. Brongo S, Nicoletti GF, La Padula S, et al. Use of lipofilling for the treatment of severe burn outcomes. Plast Reconstr Surg 2012;130(2):374e–6e.

38. Huang SH, Wu SH, Lee SS, et al. Fat grafting in burn scar alleviates neuropathic pain via anti-inflammation effect in scar and spinal cord. PLoS One 2015;10(9):e0137563.

39. Fredman R, Edkins RE, Hultman CS. Fat grafting for neuropathic pain after severe burns. Ann Plast Surg 2016;76(Suppl 4):S298–303.

40. Alessandri-Bonetti M, Egro FM, Persichetti P, et al. The role of fat grafting in alleviating neuropathic pain: a critical review of the literature. Plast Reconstr Surg Glob Open 2019;7(5):e2216.

41. Gal S, Ramirez JI, Maguina P. Autologous fat grafting does not improve burn scar appearance: a prospective, randomized, double-blinded, placebo-controlled, pilot study. Burns 2017;43(3):486–9.

42. Samadi P, Sheykhhasan M, Khoshinani HM. The Use of platelet-rich plasma in aesthetic and regenerative medicine: a Comprehensive review. Aesthetic Plast Surg 2019;43(3):803–14.

43. Zheng W, Zhao DL, Zhao YQ, et al. Effectiveness of platelet rich plasma in burn wound healing: a systematic review and meta-analysis. J Dermatolog Treat 2022;33(1):131–7.

44. Picard F, Hersant B, Bosc R, et al. Should we use platelet-rich plasma as an adjunct therapy to treat "acute wounds," "burns," and "laser therapies": a review and a proposal of a quality criteria checklist for further studies. Wound Repair Regen 2015;23(2):163–70.

45. Carter MJ, Fylling CP, Parnell LKS. Use of platelet rich plasma gel on wound healing: a systematic review and meta-analysis. Eplasty 2011;11:e38.

46. Kakudo N, Kushida S, Kusumoto K. Platelet-rich plasma: the importance of platelet separation and concentration. Plast Reconstr Surg 2009;123(3):1135–6.

47. Gonchar IV, Lipunov AR, Afanasov IM, et al. Platelet rich plasma and growth factors cocktails for diabetic foot ulcers treatment: State of art developments and future prospects. Diabetes Metab Syndr 2018;12(2):189–94.

48. Pallua N, Wolter T, Markowicz M. Platelet-rich plasma in burns. Burns 2010;36(1):4–8.

49. Maghsoudi H, Nezami N, Mirzajanzadeh M. Enhancement of burn wounds healing by platelet dressing. Int J Burns Trauma 2013;3(2):96–101.

50. Marck RE, Gardien KLM, Stekelenburg CM, et al. The application of platelet-rich plasma in the treatment of deep dermal burns: a randomized, double-blind, intra-patient controlled study. Wound Repair Regen 2016;24(4):712–20.

51. Dai Z, Lou X, Shen T, et al. Combination of ablative fractional carbon dioxide laser and platelet-rich plasma treatment to improve hypertrophic scars: a retrospective clinical observational study. Burns Trauma 2021;9. tkab016.

52. Tenna S, Cogliandro A, Barone M, et al. Comparative study using autologous fat grafts Plus platelet-rich plasma with or without fractional CO_2 laser Resurfacing in treatment of Acne scars: analysis of outcomes and satisfaction with FACE-Q. Aesthetic Plast Surg 2017;41(3):661–6.

53. Nita AC, Orzan OA, Filipescu M, et al. Fat graft, laser CO_2 and platelet-rich-plasma synergy in scars treatment. J Med Life 2013;6(4):430–3.